21 Things to Know Before Starting an Ashtanga Yoga Practice

Claudia Azula Altucher

ISBN 10: 1461147743
ISBN-13: 978-1461147749

DEDICATION

To James, I love you

CONTENTS

FOREWORD, BY A BEGINNER

Before I even met Claudia (on our very first date) I knew that she was into yoga and that yoga was her life. For me this was sexy.

In my feeble understanding of what "yoga" meant I knew that Claudia was going to be healthy (or at least making a serious attempt at living a healthy life). I knew that she probably cared how she looked (don't all yogis look beautiful and sexy, I thought?) and I knew that she probably had a spiritual side to her quest for a better life.

I was right on all counts. Then, towards the end of our first date, Claudia said: "so when do you start yoga?"

Whoah! Let me get back to you on that one.

But it was true, I needed to live a healthier life myself. We started dating and I knew I had to keep up. I started working out in a gym with a trainer. I was doing weights. But I was reading Claudia's blog and I was getting attracted to some of the philosophical aspects.

"James is a yogi" Claudia would tell her friends, "but he doesn't know it yet." And everyone would laugh. Me, most of all.

But then I got on the mat in August, 2010. Then we went to India in January 2011 and I started studying more intensively. I got into not only the physical practice but I was reading every book I could find on the spiritual practice. I felt my life improving.

My only regret now: is that I hadn't read this book and started sooner. The only problem with that is that this book didn't exist until today. Fortunately, you don't have that problem

James Altucher

ACKNOWLEDGMENTS

I bow to the lotus feet of the Teacher, Sharath Jois, of Mysore, India, current head of the Ashtanga Yoga Research Institute

And to his mother Saraswathi Rangaswamy, and her brother Manju Jois who carry the light of Ashtanga yoga by teaching all over the world

And to their Teacher before, Sri Krishna Pattabhi Jois, who said: *"Do Your Practice And All Is Coming"*

And his teacher before him, Sri Tirumalai Krishnamacharya, who said: *"Propagate Yoga Wisely"*

And his Teacher before him, Sri Ramamohan Brahmachari

And to all the teachers and gurus that came before them.

May this book be a channel for their wisdom to reach further students. May the world become a more peaceful place as a result. May we all be well.

ONE: WELCOME AND AN INTRODUCTION

May we all practice Ashtanga Yoga which brings peace to our minds and to the world.
Sharath Jois, NYC, April of 2011

Within just a few years the practice of Ashtanga Yoga has made me physically, emotionally, and mentally healthier. It is with deep gratitude and excitement that I set out to write this book in the spirit of sharing.

I am a beginner, which by Ashtanga Yoga standards means I have not practiced daily asanas (poses) –six times a week-, non-stop, for over 10, 12, 15, 30, 50 or 70 years. Depending on whom you talk to you will get a different point of view on what being a beginner means. I find that we are all beginners unless we have practiced steadily for a very long time, and in this tradition a long time means long.

I only discovered the Ashtanga Vinyasa Yoga style of Pattabhi Jois in 2004.

I am scared of writing this book. I am scared that I do not have 40 years of experience nor know how to speak Sanskrit. I am afraid because I cannot chant all of the Yoga Sutras from memory or fully place both legs behind my neck.

Yet, it is exactly the hunger produced by the fact that I am a beginner that inspires me to write it right now, before I cross that line that turns me into a more experienced practitioner or someone who just does not remember what it is like to get started.

I am telling you all of this for two reasons 1) so that you know, and 2) so that you know what to expect. This book is intended as a guide, a resource, and a conversation.

When I first started practicing I always wished I had a handbook that directed me and gave me pointers as of where to start, what to focus on first, who to ask the questions I had, how to go about those first practices, whether to travel to Mysore or not, how much would my life change? I wanted an overview or a guide.

Recently someone who has been attracted to this practice asked at the blog if I could provide such a guide because it all "felt very intimidating from the perspective of a beginner". I completely related. That is how this book was born. It is the book I wished I had, and I felt inspired to write it.

I noticed that sometimes advanced students - people who have been practicing for, say, 15 or more years- tend to forget the struggles of getting used to a whole new and demanding practice like this one, and although I am not a complete beginner anymore as I have been on the mat for a few years, I happen to be married to someone who is. Watching his progress and drawing from my own experience I put together these 21 points to serve as a guide for anyone who is curious about this fascinating process.

Let's get to it.

What is Yoga?

To actually understand this [the definition of yoga] in one's being is of a wholly different order. To understand words and concepts is easy, but to let the experience of yoga penetrate deep into one's heart, to realize fully what one is made of, and, finally, to establish the mind in the Self—these are very difficult

Sri K. Pattabhi Jois

Yoga happens when we can be present in this moment without the mind running a script that describes what it thinks is happening and tries to figure out what is in it for her. That is what the very first line of the Yoga Sutras of Patanjali (the bible of yoga) tells us: "Yoga is the cessation of the fluctuations of the mind". Sometimes I prefer the term delusions instead of fluctuations, it seems to bring the point home more clearly, as we go through life thinking that we know everything and that our mind can control things, when in reality we live in an eternal now, full of possibilities, and whatever we may think we know is just one point of view.

The basic translation from the Sanskrit term "yoga" tells us that it means to yoke, or to unite. So we unite body mind and spirit. The problem with this definition is that it is too broad, as in: What does that mean?

Intellectually I can understand it, but as I go down the street, how do I use the yoking idea to live a yogic life?

Sri K. Pattabhi Jois, the man who named the style *Ashtanga* (which means eight limbs) says in his book *Yoga Mala* that yoga is: "a path we follow by which we can attain something" and that something we are trying to attain is the "Self".

This is a great definition and as the pieces of the puzzle begin to be put together through steady practice and for a long time it will eventually make sense, however, for someone just coming into yoga it might be a bit confusing to just grasp what he means by "Self".

This Self is the part of us that is always at peace, the part that was never born and will never die, the part that is timeless, eternal, always flowing in this moment, free of compulsive thinking.

For many of us this being fully present is not possible right away as it is stated on that first yoga sutra, the mind has too much momentum, the collective thinking has a tremendous power of hypnosis over us. And so, when just being present does not work, some of us want a path to follow, steps, guidelines, and that is where the second chapter of the yoga sutras comes handy.

Patanjali gave a very clear three point description of how we can all achieve the state of yoga. He said we can gain it by doing these three things:

- ***Accepting pain as help for purification*** – this is where the physical aspects of yoga practice come from. And don't worry the pain implied is the good kind of pain.

- ***Studying of spiritual books***.

- ***Surrendering to the Supreme being***.

The actual state of yoga that we will attain is what Pattabhi Jois was trying to tell us, the identification with the Self rather than with our name or our possessions, titles, position in the world.

That not being enough Patanjali went on to elaborate further and came up with eight steps, or eight limbs, also in this chapter two. These are practices that we can do daily, in every aspect of life, from waking up in the morning to purifying the body to breathing deeply to finding silence and practice concentration. The eight limbs of yoga are called Ashtanga in Sanskrit (ashto means eight, anga means limbs). The system of yoga designed by Pattabhi Jois is based on the Yoga Sutras, but his style in particular is known as the Ashtanga Vinyasa Yoga to differentiate it.

To Me:

I noticed that all definitions of yoga written by masters only begin to make sense after a while, after one tarts participating in the journey of the practice. It is one thing to talk about it from the mental plane but a completely different story to get on a mat, sweat and see the results happening for ourselves, in real terms. In that spirit, let's get started with the parts that we can actually get our hands on.

A Very Short Account on How Ashtanga Yoga Started

A century ago, there lived a sage called Yogeshwara Ramamohan Brahmachari, a master yogi and teacher rumored to live in the mountains beyond Nepal at the foot of Mount Kailash.   One day, a young man by the name Tirumalai Krishnamacharya reached him after walking for two and half months and to study with him.

Krishnamacharya spent seven and a half years studying the Yoga Sutras of Patanjali, learning asanas –yoga poses- and pranayama –breathing extension exercises- and studying the therapeutic aspects of yoga. He was also made to memorize the whole of the Yoga Kuruntha –an ancient text believed to be lost after it was eaten by ants.

When Krishnamacharya finished his studies with Sri Ramamohan he asked how much he should pay, as it was the custom, but Ramamohan did not want money in return for his teachings. Instead he told Krishnamacharya to go out into the world, take a wife, raise children and be a teacher of yoga.

He did. In the process He attracted several students who in turn became very famous. The list includes:

- Sri Krishna Pattabhi Jois
- B.K.S Iyengar

- Srivatsa Ramaswami
- A.G. Mohan
- T.K.V. Desikachar (his son)
- Indra Devi

In 1927, at the age of 12, <u>Krishna Pattabhi Jois</u> attended a lecture by Krishnamacharya and liked it so much that he became his student the very next day. He remained with him for two years. Even at that young age he would wake up early, go to his practice and then to school, his parents never knew.

In 1930, at the tender age of 15 Jois ran away from home to study Sanskrit and with only 2 rupees to his name, but Krishnamacharya had left town. It was not until two years later that they were reunited when Krishnamacharya returned to Mysore.

At that time the Maharaja of Mysore became the patron of Krishnamacharya and established a yoga shala –studio- for him in the palace. Krishnamacharya remained with Jois until 1941, then left for Madras.

In 1948 with the help of students, Jois purchased a home in the Mysore section of town called Lakshmipuram, where he lived with his wife and three children Saraswathi, Manju and Ramesh.

He held a teaching position in yoga at the Sanskrit College of Maharaja from 1937 to 1973 when he left to devote himself fully to teach yoga at his yoga shala. In 1948, he established the Ashtanga Yoga Research Institute.

In 1964, a Belgian named André Van Lysebeth spent two months with Jois learning the primary and intermediate asanas of the Ashtanga Vinyasa Yoga system. Not long afterwards, van Lysebeth wrote a book called *J'apprends le Yoga* (1967) in which he mentioned Jois and included his address. This marked the beginning of westerners coming to Mysore to study yoga.

Jois wrote his only book, *Yoga Mala*, in Kannada in 1958. The book was published in English in 1999.

Jois continued to teach at the Ashtanga Yoga Research Institute in Mysore, now located in the neighborhood of Gokulam, with his only daughter Saraswathi and his grandson Sharath until May 18, 2009 when he died aged 93.

Both Sharath and Saraswathi continue teaching at the shala in Mysore and in tours throughout the world. Manju Jois also teaches in the United States and internationally.

Sharath Jois is the current director of the Ashtanga Yoga Research institute and he will be mentioned quite a bit throughout the book.

TWO: DO YOUR PRACTICE AND ALL IS COMING

The date on the receipt for my first purchase of an Ashtanga Yoga instructional DVD -for the primary series- is mid-2005. I had been toying with the idea of committing to the practice by following along video tapes that I borrowed from the New York Public library, mostly Richard Freeman's instructions. Even though my practice began to get some traction relatively fast, I could not get myself to practice every day, it seemed like a lot.

I was too shy to go to a studio, I needed to know at least some of the poses (or so I told myself) before I would venture into a classroom setting. It took me still two more years from the day I received that DVD, until I finally committed to start a daily practice, non-stop, six times a week and with a teacher.

It is important to know that Ashtanga Yoga is a life-time process and not a *get rich quick* thing. Far from it. It is good to take it one thing at the time. You may also want to look at the resources and see what resonates with you to begin your own exploration when you are ready. The one thing I can tell you is that it gets more and more interesting by the day, especially when the effort begins to bear fruit and positive changes in life begin to manifest.

On my first trip to Mysore in early 2008 while talking to a very advanced student about how I felt terrified about poses like: _kurmasana_ –one of the most difficult poses of the primary series where the legs attempt to go behind the head- he said to me: "give it three years, and the body will open". Three years! What?!

That is how Ashtanga students think, in terms of years if not decades. Opening a body that has been sitting in a desk or living a sedentary life takes time, and it's OK, there is no rush, nowhere to go but inwards.

"Asana" is the practice of the poses of yoga and it is important to start here, to get on the mat and do what you can. To get used to it. It might be that you get to it only one or two times a week in the beginning. That is fine, most of us started that way, me included as you now know.

It takes a lot to commit to a daily routine, but I find that the practice itself contains within it the seeds that will sprout, in due time, into something we do every day. Believe it or not, getting on the mat six times per week eventually happens as we begin to notice the benefits of the practice and prefer them over our own old routines.

Suddenly we notice that we feel better on the days we practice and not so good on the days we do not. We then start re-arranging our lives so that practice can take precedent.

Maybe we wake up earlier, maybe we join a Mysore program, then we make friends in the yoga studio, and we create a community. Gradually we are immersed in this new world, our life begins to change for the better and we start reaping the benefits of the deep breathing, the time to ourselves, and the healing nuances of the practice.

So do not worry, get on the mat - all the rest will come.

Focusing On Asana Practice First

99% Practice, 1% Theory
Sri K. Pattabhi Jois

The first step in Ashtanga Vinyasa Yoga is to learn what is called the primary series of asanas. This word: "asana/s", will be always used from now on meaning yoga poses.

At least in the beginning just work on getting on the mat as much as possible and doing what you can. If you have access to a good teacher then you are very lucky as she or he will guide you. If you don't then look at the resources at the end of the book for good DVDs to start at home with. Just keep in mind that it is recommended to go to a teacher as soon as possible. Some people can learn on their own but in my observations of hundreds and hundreds of practitioners and what they had to say, a teacher is always the best way to learn, especially because this practice is so demanding and it has so many elements (breathing, looking points, internal locks).

In my own case I was surprised to find out how many poses I was doing with wrong alignment and how my breathing was out of sorts when I practiced at home. An experienced teacher can help us go deeper into the practice, and faster.

The practice of asana is the doorway into yoga, and this is especially true for us in the westerner world, where so many things compete for our attention. Just having an hour or ninety minutes to ourselves where we can quietly focus on our breath and body is revolutionary.

You probably heard that yoga is not just the poses. That is true, it is not just that, but the poses are the beginning, they are the passport to becoming healthy. It all starts at the level of how our body is feeling, and how healthy we are.

Sharath Jois, recently said at a New York City conference that: *The practice starts with asana because it is a strong body that will focus our mind and end the delusions.* That is why the emphasis is completely on surrendering to, and achieving, a daily asana practice. Then keeping it up for a long, long time.

The first two of the eight limbs of yoga are called *yama* and *niyama*, (or the five abstentions and the five observances) and they are difficult to master.

Take for example the very first *yama*: "*ahimsha*" or *non-violence* has so many subtleties that it might require a lifetime of work to come to terms with it. We may all think that we are not violent. When I started practicing I was convinced that I was not violent at all, but little by little I discovered that I was.

Violence has subtle levels. For example, few weekends ago I visited department store, tried on a dress, and looked in the mirror. Out of nowhere I heard my mind begin to shot as if it was a gun telling me how horrible I looked, how my stomach was out of proportion, how I was old, and how I looked hideous. Years of yoga and perhaps some wisdom that comes with time, helped me identify that this was just a thought-pattern and that I had the choice to believe it or not. I eventually let it go, but this is very much a violent act of the mind.

Some practitioners want to hurry and get into very advanced poses very quickly, and in the process injure themselves. I have read and heard many stories of this happening, and when you think it through you realize that violence against ourselves can be a sneaky thing. It can almost pass unnoticed as we push harder to get ahead or to try to look cool by showing off our dexterity.

As you get started, it might be helpful to just think of being ethical, as in: working at not being violent, or refraining from stealing –including paper clips in the office-, adopting an attitude of contentment, observing the places where you speak your truth and where you tell lies, especially to yourself.

A strong body and clear mind are needed to discriminate to an extent in which we might be able to reach all of these limbs of yoga, and consequently be of good use to society. We start with asana practice, and then we begin to pay attention to our daily actions. All comes.

Curiosity for the other branches will be awakened, but the daunting task of trying to grasp everything at once could discourage us from practice. I suspect this is why Pattabhi Jois said his famous: ***99% practice 1% theory***. We cannot get into the deeper limbs of yoga like, say, for example pranayama (breathing extension), if our bodies are not healed and strong.

Asana comes in first as a blessing and as a way to restore our bodies to their original blue-print. The daily practice on the mat makes us stronger and gives us the nervous system that is required to withstand the energy that comes with the upper branches in the tree of yoga which include for example, the ability to concentrate single-minded on one object for long periods of time.

Remember that we are talking about attaining full peace and enlightenment, about transforming our lives so that we become kind beings with full discrimination, living entities that speak and act truth with no delusions. Humans who are present and not acting from pre-conceived judgments.

Things have got to change somewhat to accommodate such powerful energies, and a strong and healthy body is the foundation.

Once we have practiced for a while then we can start thinking about *pranayama*, *pratyahara* or sense withdrawal, which is the fifth limb and leads one into *concentration* –the sixth-, *meditation* –the seventh- and *Samadhi* or enlightenment, the last limb. But first things first. Let us get on the mat and try to build that six times a week routine. Let's taste the benefits of what this change can bring, then we will move on.

It Is A Breathing Practice

Anybody can breathe. Therefore anybody can practice yoga.
T.K.V. Desikachar

The interesting thing about the primary series of Ashtanga yoga is that it never stops, it keeps you moving from the very first movement and until we rest in *savasana* – corpse pose-. All the poses are linked together by what is called *vinyasa*, or ways in which we get out of one pose and into the next. It is a little bit like a slow dance.

As you start to practice the primary series, make your breathing the first priority, slow down if you have to, make sure to breathe slow and steady, long breaths. When you think you are breathing slow, think slower.

The second priority is to coordinate the movement to the breath, easy does it.

The breathing is done in a very specific way which Sharath calls *deep breathing with sound*. We make a noise as we inhale and as we exhale that resembles Darth Vader's breath. You can try it right now, think Vader and then take a long inhale, you will see that the breath comes in slower and that you make a sound, exhale in the same way, there you go, you are doing it.

What happens is that we contract the glottis so that the air is inhaled and exhaled in a controlled and slow way. One interesting thing about yogis is that they measure their longevity in breaths rather than in years, and when you make this kind of shift in your thinking then each breath becomes a precious thing, every one of them is tasted and elongated. We become connoisseurs of the breath. We do this consciously during yoga practice, we make the breath long and steady, and the sound we make is, as master teacher Krishnamacharya would say, *like the hissing of a serpent*.

Over time your breathing will become smooth, long and controlled. The breathing is the basic support of the practice. Over the years we build our stamina and strength on smoother and longer breaths.

Every movement in the series of Ashtanga yoga is intimately paired with a breathing movement, nothing is left to chance. Arms go up on the inhale (for example) and then we float them down into a standing forward bend on the exhale, it is a dance. However, as the series progress we may feel as if the air is not enough, we may get fatigued, especially in the beginning.

I was just talking to someone who recently started practicing and was reminded of how at first it is OK to add extra breaths and aim to get the flow of the sequence right. Sometimes it is not possible to maintain a steady breath as we start adding the jumping back and through in between each one of the poses. Extra breaths may be needed. In cases like this, the good eye of an experienced teacher can guide and direct us. When in doubt however, always make the breath the priority.

The Primary Series is called Yoga Therapy -*Chikitsa*- because it slowly sends air to parts of our body where perhaps it never reached before, it tones the body, cleanses the internal organs (especially those of digestion and elimination) and makes use of muscles we had no idea we had. Our body needs ventilating after decades of pollution (physical, emotional, mental, spiritual pollution). Breathing via Ashtanga Vinyasa yoga ventilates the whole body.

When I first started practicing in a studio I noticed that they offered "*Half*-Primary Led Classes". If you can find these, and the teacher clicks with you, then you are in luck.

Half Led Primary Classes are shorter versions of the primary series, not too daunting, not so long, and usually going all the way but not further than *Navasana* (the boat pose) which is the pose that comes after the twists. The good thing is that you get to learn the counts, you benefit from the group energy, you begin to learn how to breathe, and hey! You are practicing.

"Drishti" Or Gaze. Where To Focus The Eyes In Each Pose

Every asana in the primary series (and all six series) has a focus point, either we look at the hand, or the tip of the nose (alongside the tip, no eye-crossing) or the left, or the right, and so on.

Your teacher will point to you which way the gazing has to go or you can find out by doing research from books in the resource chapter. Do not worry too much in the beginning, just be aware of it. Slowly it will all come together like the pieces of a puzzle, and over years of practice.

The Drishtis of the practice are:

1. Tip of the nose: Asagrai

2. The navel: Nabi Chakra

3. The hand: Hastagrai

4. The toes: Padayorgrai

5. The thumbs: Angusta Ma Dyai

6. Up to the sky: Urdhva / Antara Drishti

7. Far to the right or to the left: Parsva

8. The third eye: Ajna Chakra / Broomadhya

When in doubt, you cannot go wrong if you look alongside the line of the tip of your nose, but it is a good practice to learn the different focus points eventually.

Bandhas: How We Prevent Energy Leaks

Bandhas are internal locks. The most important one at first is the mulabandha or root chakra lock. This is done by contracting the area of the perineum. Pattabhi Jois was known for saying *"tighten your anus"*, and for maintaining that you should actually contract this area of the body most of the time.

The contraction of the area of the perineum is used to summon our energy, direct it upwards, and prevent it from leaking. When we lock the root portion of the body we ensure that the base of our energy source is active and connected. Not only that, we also connect with the energy of the legs, which I was surprised to find out, I could forget when the poses would get difficult.

There is a second Bandha called "Uddyiana badha" in the area of the navel which pulls the energy upwards. The idea is that once the energy is harnessed from the root it is sent upwards.

Be aware of the root bandha but at least at first do not worry too much. Just learning the standing sequence of the primary series is enough work. Keep in mind that there is a basic lock that needs to happen but if you forget it at first it's OK. Your teacher will remind you from time to time, and eventually it will become part of your practice.

Tristasana: When The Practice Begins To Bear Fruit

After a long time of steady practice one may be lucky enough to have all the elements of the practice come together while on the mat. The poses will feel strong, the body cleansed and supple, the gaze completely directed towards its point of attention and the breathing deep and smooth, hissing like a serpent, reaching every corner of the body, revitalizing it. A meditative state comes as a result when all of this comes together, and this is what is known as *tristasana*.

Where is the bandha component in all of this? Recently a student at the Ashtanga Yoga Research Institute (AYRI) in Mysore asked Sharath that question and he reminded us all that bandhas, Guru used to say, must be engaged at all times, at least the root bandha, and that is why it does not make it into the tristasana, although of course, on that perfect, grace-filled practice, all bandhas would be engaged appropriately, naturally.

How long would that take? This is a question that used to lurk in my mind when I started practicing. Here is Tirumalai Krishnamacharya himself answering from his book Yoga Makaranda:

After all the activities and movements of the mind cease, the mind ... becomes steady. Until it develops this steadiness, we do not obtain any benefits from it. Until the mind is made to remain steady, all the time spent on this pursuit will be wasted and we will not receive any benefits from actions performed by a shaky mind. As a result, some might ask, if spending time on yoga might not initially produce any benefit then why should one practice it?.... "No accomplishment or achievement is possible without effort" is a great saying. "

What Does "All Is Coming" Mean?

Mastery of yoga is really measured by how it influences our day-to-day living, how it enhances our relationships, how it promotes clarity and peace of mind.
T.K.V. Desikachar

I have always wondered about what the "all" in: "*Do your practice and all is coming*" meant. I can only speak from my experience but I will say that the best way to know that your practice is working is that your life get better.

If I had to describe the cycle of how the "all" comes about, it would go something like this:

The daily asana practice begins to cleanse our bodies in a deep and profound way, so much so that our cycles of food-intake, rest, and elimination become cleaner, efficient, and stable. Also, as we are getting on the mat every day, our body finds new ways to release toxins that have accumulated over years, through sweating, twisting, inversions, etc.

As a result of these new healthier habits the body becomes stronger, leaner, and supple which in turn helps the mind become more focused and efficient in its thinking process.

Because of the new gained clarity we make better choices and begin to use our energy more effectively in all areas of our lives. For example, we get clear about who are our friends and who just pretend to be, who is a positive influence and who steals our energy instead. We get clear about how we are using our sexual energy, we pay more attention to our creativity and our instincts, we become more in-tune with our own spirit or our Self.

As a consequence we get better results in our lives which ultimately lead to better living conditions, better surroundings and better energies around us.

Not only that but the deep breathing results in us slowing down a little, perhaps skipping a bit and thinking before starting or continuing with an argument we know will be going nowhere. These extra little silences help us notice things that we never noticed before. We become more aware of coincidences in life, perhaps we start taking them as cues from universal intelligence directing us to go in a certain direction or to not do some other thing. And so we act accordingly. Faith and trust develops. We feel better and an overall well-being flows through us.

All the things we want begin to come to us provided they help us on the way to our own truth. There is the *all*.

All those things we think we want but are not really relevant for our spiritual development somehow either disappear from our radar or fade away.

The ultimate paradox is that after a long time of dedicated and focused practice we start wanting less things, even though they become more accessible.

But It's Hard And It Hurts

Right pain is usually felt as a gradual lengthening and strengthening feeling and must be differentiated from wrong pain, which is often a sharp and sudden cautionary feeling telling us we have gone too far beyond our present abilities.
B.K.S. Iyengar

Recently I conducted a poll at the blog asking whether people though that the popularity of Ashtanga Yoga was increasing, decreasing or they just were not sure. 56% though that it was increasing. This was not a big poll, and it was conducted in an Ashtanga-focused type of blog, so that may not have been so surprising, but what did surprise me was the conversation sparkled in the comments over the reasons why its popularity might be rising, yes, but not so fast: the majority of commentators said that people consider it "hard". I get it.

When I first started practicing Ashtanga Yoga I would switch between Mark Darby's primary series DVD, and Richard Freeman's intermediate series DVD. Monday for Darby's, Tuesday for Freeman's.

I had never done Ashtanga before, so I thought I could breeze through the different series at will and make my own routines without consulting anyone. I thought kapotasana (a very deep backbend of intermediate) as well as other contorted poses would not be that hard. Was I deluded? Completely!

When I see James (a beginner and my husband) come out of one of the led classes expressionless other than using enough muscle to say: "*brutal!*", then it looks hard. Let's also point out that he, just like me, has been bitten by the "wanting to do it all at once" bug. It's in the air.

Then I wonder: who, initially, among us follows the system exactly as intended and with a good teacher? In the way intended we practice with a teacher, in a Mysore room, learning one pose at the time, moving along only when ready. We also take a led class or two each week to clarify and clean up the counting, the breathing, sequencing, etc.

We are never to be moved to the next pose until we can somewhat "master" the one we are on which is determined by the watchful eye of someone more experienced than us. There is energetic intelligence behind this, we do not practice the next pose, even if we may think it is easy, because that way we have sufficient energy to concentrate on what we have, which more often than not is plenty enough.

I am one of those people who wants everything fast, or at least I did. I wanted those advanced poses like the difficult inversions of the intermediate series. Hey! I even had an Excel chart outlining how I wanted my practice to unfold and when I would learn some of the poses. You can clearly see how my mind tends to take over from time to time, and how the practice informs me that I am not present, but rather making calculations, giving thoughts a much bigger place than they deserve, a slave of my mind rather than someone that uses it for good.

One commentator on the blog said: "*it requires getting over the idea that it will be boring*". I actually never had this problem, the asana part of Ashtanga was never boring to me, but I can relate to how the repetition can be unsettling for a mind used to watching three screens at once, or multitasking, or having a high frequency type of job for a living.

Yes, this practice demands a change of pace. And if you think about it, slowing down is really not that bad.

Another commentator suggested that starting an Ashtanga yoga asana practice could be compared to giving birth, one of those painful moments that are forgotten and even romanticized later on. I have never given birth, but have heard that story, all I know is that the original pain that I felt was labeled in my mind as "good pain", the pain of purification, the pain that was cleansing my system. And I always remembered and was directed by teachers to never force, to just work with finding the edge.

Someone else with a home practice mentioned how he finally came to find a good teacher, and although he only sees her when on tour it is a key part of his practice. And I have to say that yes, finding a good teacher that will go along, respect our limitations, and work with our mental fluctuations is critical. Not everyone is that lucky.

I will confess to one thing that I found very hard in the beginning. It was the moment when you are practicing and the instant before you start to sweat. I hated that moment, I did not like getting wet and dirty, I did not like to feel the burn. And that is actually the purification part, that is the moment where the healing is happening. I had a resistance to the cleansing. I find that very curious. The one thing I found helpful with this was to always bathe before and after practice. Before because a warm bath or shower loosens the body and makes it feel refreshed, it also creates a sort of ritual around the daily routine. After, because I never wanted to carry around all those toxins that were released during the practice.

So, these are the thoughts gathered around what the hard parts in Ashtanga Yoga asana are:

- The *boredom* factor
- The *pushing* to go faster because we all want to be good on day one, OK maybe not you, but I did (although not any more)
- The *sweating*. Who likes to sweat?
- The enormous *commitment*.
- Having the *stamina* to remain with the practice until it becomes a discipline that grounds us.
- Keeping *motivated*. Especially if we do not have a good teacher nearby or cannot make it to Mysore
- Before starting the practice: dealing with the *perception that it is hard*
- *Finding a good teacher* that will help us find our edge and slow our mental fanatical desire to go further. Also, avoiding a teacher that could hurt us.

Finding a good teacher is difficult. I agree with that. Whether it be in person or online, or through workshops, coming across the right soul, that is hard indeed.

But can you see how all the other points in the list reside in the mind of the beholder?

It may not be easy, but it is actually not hard, not if we follow the traditional method, not if we can get out of the way and surrender. Not if we just let the mind do its thing and still get on the front of the mat, then take that first breath.

> *Body is not stiff. Mind is.*
> Sri Krishna Pattabhi Jois

THREE: 21 THINGS I WISH I KNEW BEFORE I STARTED PRACTICING ASHTANGA YOGA

Vinyasa means breathing and movement system. For each movement there is one breath. In this way all asanas are assigned a certain number of vinyasas.

From the KPJAYI website

From the very beginning I was completely intrigued by Ashtanga. Starting with its brutal schedule, its lack of poetry (no: "feel the earth's energy flow through you" ever heard in a class), and mythological superstition, as in: no new poses to be taught on Tuesdays because it is ruled by Mars which is the God of war.

What I loved immediately was the sense of independence that it gave me. "Finally!" I thought to myself, a very specific approach to practice which, in spite of having a lot in common with all other styles, has one single element that makes it stand out: it is done as a self-practice where each student arrives in their own time and does his or her practice while the teacher comes around to adjusts individually.

Known as the *Mysore style* (due to its birth-place in India), I ventured into it with an open heart one April fool's day. Looking back there are a few things I wish someone had whispered in my ear as I embarked on such a colossal journey, these are 21 of the most notorious:

1. – The Breathing

Breathing is the most important and relevant thing within the practice. As one embarks on the primary series the first curious thing is that there is no pause, one keeps breathing and flowing from one asana to the next and the body is constantly moving following exact prescribed movements while riding the breath.

It is not uncommon in the beginning to go to the extremes, either get out of breath, or to turn into a "respirator" (as I like to call it) by loudly forcing it.

I have myself been in both extremes and either breathed loudly and fast trying to catch up with the movement or not breathed at all in days where I wanted to be numb and avoid life in general.

It is a practice for that reason; we aim towards the middle path. The breathing of the Mysore practice is as important as it is difficult to understand.

The amount of push and sound need be only as much as is required to generate heat, focus, and reach the edge of each asana, then transcend it. One good suggestion I heard from a teacher once was that I was the one that needed to hear the breath, not everyone else.

2.- Hot and Hard

Mysore classes can get really hot, especially when the rooms are crowded, it is summer, or you are in a tropical place. Sweat is profuse when the practice starts to get deep and the purification process of the first series kicks in. Perspiration goes hand in hand with daily practice and it is best to make peace with it, and do some research on good deodorants.

3.-Weight Release Happens

Coming into the practice I noticed how most advanced practitioners had beautiful and balanced bodies. I wanted that. I learned eventually that the practice might not turn me into a runway model, but that instead it would return my body to its original blue-print, which it did because of the intensity of the asana and as soon as a momentum was reached.

For example: I learned very quickly that to do the deep twists in the middle of the first series (*Marichasanas*) I needed an empty stomach, a very empty one, and so having the last meal before 7 PM at night became an easy routine. Through the health momentum of yoga I actually released 30 pounds.

4.-"Ladies Holidays" and: Do I Shower Before Practice? After? Or Both?

Ladies holidays refers to the days in which a woman is menstruating; I have seen women who never take rest during these days and women who take two or even three days off. In the end it is a very personal choice. In India the suggestion is to take three full days of rest, but I have found that practitioners in the west seem to have a very different opinion. Most women pay no attention to these special days and practice anyway; they make some adjustments (like no inversions) but do not stop. In my own case I learned that it is best to take rest and I do, I also welcome it.

As per the showering, the tacit agreement is that everyone showers both before and after. I used to think that if I was going to "exercise and sweat" then what was the point of pre-showering anyway? That is, until I happened to practice next to a fellow that smelled. That changed everything. Now I shower before and after, even if I practice alone.

Also, showering pre-practice prepares the body and can at times help loosen it. Showering post practice is a blessing as it cleans all the impurities that were brought to the surface by the exertions.

5.-Should You Forget a Pose in the Sequence...

About five months into my own practice one day I skipped a pose, did not notice and kept going. Later on the teacher came over and had me go back and repeat from where I had skipped about seven poses earlier. Ouch! I learned the lesson.

On the other hand I also started to become "shala smart" and hide my mistakes if they ever happened again, which they did, and to pay more and more attention every day, until the practice became a bit automatic, which is in itself another danger. Not all teachers make people go back and repeat, but I feel it was a very good learning experience for me.

6.-Pose Advancement Anxiety

I did not anticipate when I started that I would crave and have internal battles over wanting more poses, reaching second series, advancing, moving. My explosive intent to keep growing, show off, be better, is one that my mind has very ingrained. Then I noticed that the desire would go in cycles, sometimes I would want more sometimes I would not want anything. I would not say I am completely surrendered to the process by now, but at least I am laughing at it a bit more.

The fastest way to get the next pose is to perfect the ones you already have.
Sharath Jois, Mysore 2011

7.-The Addiction

The practice is addictive, or, perhaps a better expression is "habit forming". Once you start practicing you will crave it and will practice everywhere you go, in your brother's terrace, an airborne plane (in the kitchen area until the kick you out), behind the airport counter or just all out in full display while waiting for the next plane out of Dubai.

I did all of those.

8.-It's OK to Say No to Adjustments

Until trust is established with a teacher it is not only OK but also healthy to keep strong boundaries when it comes to adjustments. In a good way, of course, no need to be rude. A good teacher will always observe your practice first before attempting to change things.

It is important to always respect our bodies and what we know about them.

It is also good to be careful not to fall too much on the other side, as adjustments are useful, and certain poses -I am pretty sure- are impossible without them, for example Supta Kurmasana, in which the legs go behind the neck, which takes not just one adjustment but years of them.

9.-Why Rest on Moon Days?

The practice happens six times a week and this is a plus as it leaves very little room for laziness or hesitation. The only days of rest are Saturdays, ladies holidays, and new/full moon days. Why is that? There are many theories. One of them that makes sense to me comes from a senior teacher from Encinitas called Tim Miller. He maintains that our bodies are mostly water which in turn, just as the oceans are influenced by the ties and cycles of the moon.

A new moon is then compared to the end of a breathing cycle -the end of the exhale- where we normally pause and then breath in, while the full moon would be the equivalent of the top of the inhale when, with filled lungs, we briefly pause to start the cycle all over again.

10.-Conversations Get Technical

Some yogis are very much into the asana part, and you will encounter them. They are fascinating people to talk to because you start to get very precise about what happens and what is needed in a pose. I am grateful to have a few yogis in my life who love discussing every single detail. You will notice that not only do you learn the Sanskrit words for the poses but you will also learn the names of the muscles you use in each of them (do you know where your psoas is?). You might also being to talk quite a bit about your anus and the perineum.

11.-Led Classes Are Useful. Fun? Maybe Not So Much

Because the practice is self-directed the tradition provides one led (or guided) class per week. Not all studios subscribe to this but more and more are catching on. The good thing about it is that you get to learn the true count and it helps with cleaning up any extra movements you may have "creatively" added, I know I do from time to time.

So they are useful, but for me not so much fun as the count, for example, could be slow in a pose that you may not like. It happens. We learn surrender.

This comes useful for life in general as throughout the day we are bound to encounter uncomfortable situations, and learning to breathe through them is a good practice.

12.-Cult Accusations

Yes, you might be the target of accusations of having joined a cult, which is sweet really, and partly true, as there are a few practitioners out there who can get very fanatic about it, which brings me to...

13.-Keeping a Healthy Sense of Humor

It is a challenge to maintain a sense of humor, an attitude of detachment, and to admit that hey! other practices also work well. I encounter yoga practitioners all the time and all over the world, each has their own preference, nobody can tell someone else what will work for them, it is a very personal journey, whatever helps us become more peaceful and more present is it.

14.-Bandhas

I am still not sure I will ever understand the full story behind bandhas. They are basically internal locks which one engages during asana practice; one is in the area of the perineum (moola bandha), and: "Tighten the anus" is a phrase you need to be prepared to hear.

The other one is in the area of the navel (uddiyana bandha). Their main purpose is to prevent energy from leaking out of the body and induce it to flow upwards through the chakras and eventually enlighten us.

All very interesting but a life time of work to understand at a visceral level. By the way there is a third bandha (in the area of the throat) and an ongoing debate around weather it should be engaged during practice or not, but that is material for another book.

15-Change in Social Habits and in Life

Not everyone enjoys going out at night with a deadline of "I need to be asleep by 9". Waking up at 5 AM on a consistent basis changes things.

16.-Going to Mysore is Recommended

Mysore (yes as in "my-sore") in Southern India is the Mecca of Ashtanga and a place of wonder. It feels like another planet, yet there is so much to see and learn there. You can visit Mysorepedia.com, a site I created where I compiled all information for it, and also for stories and photographs about the place. It is indeed something to live through, even if only once.

17.-Learning Sanskrit Happens

There is no way out, it starts with learning the names of those asanas, with wanting to understand what others are talking about, with asking what is "fill-in-the-blank-asana?" Followed by someone mimicking a pose for a response. It just happens. The beautiful thing is that it gets deeper when we realize that in the sound of Sanskrit there is more than just noise, there is magic, power.

Sanskrit happens, the sooner the better. Besides, it's pretty cool.

18.-The Yoga Sutras of Patanjali

The Yoga Sutras of Patanjali are the other side of the coin. The front side is the asana, but without the sutras they begin to feel empty. Patanjali wrote 196 short sentences which need de-coding, and that take us through all the limbs of yoga, and beyond the asanas.

This decoding is not really a mental process, each of the sentences points in the direction of the state of yoga.

Throw them into the mix and it all becomes a matrix of wisdom, the Indiana Jones journey of yoga excavation into your authentic Self begins.   The sutras clearly identify **the 8 limbs** of yoga that lead to happiness or liberation. In the end it all comes down to the opening line, yoga is the cessation of the fluctuation of the mind. Yoga is all about getting out of our own way, it is about how present we can be, how detached from what our mind tells us we should be doing, thinking, doing. A state of yoga comes when we can act from the powerful center that comes from a strong presence and no interference from precodnitionings.

19.-Indian Mythology and its Powerful Symbols

There are fantastic stories in Indian Mythology, so many that you probably won't hear them all in just one lifetime.

One, for example is that of Shiva and how he drunk the poison that was threatening to destroy the world but did not swallow it, just kept it in his throat, and that is the reason why his neck is blue.

I love the symbolism of that story because Shiva took things for what they were, he did not make a drama about it, he did not swallow the farce, he did not think about it, he just stayed with it, with full presence but not reacting, and in so doing destroyed the poison.

There are thousands of stories like this that contain deep teachings in their symbolism.

20.-Curiosity For The Other Branches

The eight limbs are marks along the territory leading to enlightenment, which so far and in my limited understanding I can only describe as eternal peace with full discrimination.

There is a deeper reality happening as we speak, a timeless wisdom and intelligence manifesting itself. We have access to all of this in this very moment, if we can get the crazy thinking to let us see it. It is difficult to see this because we are so burdened with daily life and our minds fall into intense chatter, the aim of yoga is to get in touch with the vastness, with what Rumi calls "the beloved". The upper limbs contain a map towards it.

21.-You'll Go Down The Rabbit Hole

At some point we just do, maybe we visit Mysore or we come across a very good teacher that encourages scripture reading, and we read the Yoga Sutras, or the Bhagavad Gita, or the Upanishads, and all of a sudden we find ourselves in a whole new world where the possibilities opened by yoga go far deeper than we ever dreamed of.

FOUR: A FEW REASONS WHY I CHOSE TO PRACTICE ASHTANGA YOGA AND CONTINUE TO DO SO

I will never preach or try to convince anyone of anything, but I can tell you some of the reasons why I came into Ashtanga, why it has, and how it continues work for me. There are many styles of asana practice out there, this one in particular resonated with me in a deep way, because it has:

1- Regularity and No Mind

It is practiced every day, six times a week, no questions asked, no excuses. I liked this because it gave me a tremendous sense of discipline and a focus for the day. There is also a great feeling in knowing that you have accomplished something and it is not even 9 AM. Knowing that the practice happens no matter what leaves the mind out of the equation, once it becomes a routine the mind does not even get on the way anymore, and if anything it might even cooperate in getting me to the front of the mat.

2-I Like to Travel

The practice is portable. Whenever I land, anywhere, primary series is the first thing I do, and I don't need a teacher (unless I want to go to a studio). Primary series re-aligns me, and helps in easing the jet-lag symptoms.

3- More Than a Workout

The Primary series shattered the belief I had that yoga was easy and calm or not really a workout. Just doing the standing poses of the primary series, at least in the beginning, when I first took on the practice, felt like Olympic training to me.

It is tempting to get carried away by that old saying that we will do only "what our body wants", and maybe one day we will skip that standing poses because, well, we are just not in the mood. I once heard a very senior teacher say that if it is not broken and there is no fever then we must get on the mat. That guideline goes with me everywhere and has proven very useful in those days when my mind tries to convince me not to practice.

Here is a the article written by that teacher.   In case you are reading this in paperback the link is this: http://www.centeredyoga.com/writ_body.html

4-There is More To it Than A Nice Body

When I started practicing I wanted to look good, and I noticed that most people who practice Ashtanga look really good. Their bodies seem evenly proportioned, their muscles toned but nothing stands out in a grotesque way, it is all very elegant.

However, regular practice revealed to me a much deeper sense of what yoga means, not just physically but also mentally, and spiritually. Through the body I began to notice the mental tendencies I had. This is something that continues to this day, and in every session on the mat. Being uncomfortable in a position and yet staying with it, breathing in it, is another way in which yoga helps me with much more than just keeping the body in good form, it informs me of what to do later on in life as well, when I feel uncomfortable, and I just breathe through that as well.

5-Guaranteed

It is a proven system, ask anyone who has been practicing it for a long time and you will see how much they love it and how their lives have been transformed, most likely for the better.

Besides it is a system that comes from a lineage of at least four generations of real yogis, people that woke up every morning to the practice, just like you and me do.

6-It's a Challenge

I find the challenge a blessing. Recently I heard a long-term practitioner say that finishing the second series of Ashtanga is akin to becoming an athlete. Her words resonated, Ashtanga yoga is a challenge. And it being a challenge is a blessing in disguise because our westerner mind is wired to look for one, so what better opportunity to put our natural tendencies to work with such beneficial result prospects.

7-Miracles

When we practice from the heart and sincerely we become a lot more aware of our surroundings. We notice things. Coincidences start to happen, or maybe it is because we notice them that we think they are happening. We begin to find ourselves in the right place at the right time, life becomes a thread of well-being, and we find discover we are on the path to peace and happiness, curious about all limbs and deeply immersed in a practice of health and abundance.

FIVE: THE HEALING BENEFITS OF THE PRIMARY SERIES

"The stomach is the only cause of an untimely death. There is no other reason. The dwelling place of death in the body is only the big stomach and nowhere else.
T. Krishnamacharya, in "Yoga Makaranda"

If you look at the cumulative effects of the poses of the primary series you will notice that the main focus is on clearing the digestive and elimination systems.

In his book *Yoga Mala*, Pattabhi Jois lists all of the asanas of the primary series and their benefits one by one. Looking at it you can see how all effort is directed towards making the body lean, eliminating bad fats, and clearing constipation.

For example, consider the following mentions of benefits among the postures of the primary series:

- Removes stomach bad fat: 10 mentions

- Purifies anal canal: 10 mentions

- Cures constipation: 3 mentions

- Increases or strengthens the digestive fire: 3 mentions

To begin with, the first two poses right after the opening sun salutations, *Padangusthasana* and *Padahastasana*, (standing forward bends), have the ability to dissolve the fat of the lower abdomen and purify the anal canal, kidneys and lower abdomen.

Simple standing poses like the regular and revolved triangles dissolve the fat area of the waist and bring the body into shape.

Further along the primary series there is that pose which you can see on the front cover of the book, *Utthita Hasta Padangusthasana*. This one helps with eliminating constipation, as do all the *Prasarita Padottanasanas* (A,B,C,and D).

Later on, an unsuspected boat pose, *Navasana*, purifies the anal channel and lower abdomen.

So, just as Krishnamacharya advises in that quote at the beginning of this chapter, primary series may very well be the ticket to avoiding an untimely death.

SIX: 3 SPECIFIC CASES IN WHICH YOGA HELPED ME PERSONALLY

How I Survived The Biggest Financial Crisis Of My Life

As I followed my boss through the hallway I wondered what could she possibly have to talk to me in such a rush after I had been away for five weeks in Thailand for yoga teacher training.

The sight of Celene, the Human Resources manager, clarified it all. After 10 years I was being fired. The time was early 2009.

From then on it was like a movie, I absorbed the faces of concern, the fake extra-detailed reassurance of my boss saying that it had nothing to do with my performance, the cheap talk about how this was difficult, the fear in their faces, I mean: Would I sue like everyone else does in NYC?

Would I cry? Go postal? I had, after all, mortgage payments north of 2000 dollars per month in the worst housing market of the past 30 years, a car, a yoga monthly membership, credit card debt, no family in the United States, not a penny in my pocket.

Of all the shocking situations I have lived through this one felt the most real because it had to do with the very practical technicalities of what I was going to eat the following week. With where I was going to sleep if my house was foreclosed: the YMCA? friend's couch? a shelter? Times Square?

I remember walking back into my cubicle knowing that I could go home now, that it was all over, something I had secretly desired for years.

MS Outlook showed 2127 unread messages. A form on my desk had a post it in it asking me to re-do some entry in the helpdesk database, and another asked for an explanation of a cell phone charge while in Hong Kong. I felt a burst of anger and laughed out loud. In my mind I gave them all the finger, I was now beyond all those mundane things I did not care for. I was free, powerful even.

Then of course I crashed.

Walking down Six Avenue later that morning I remember looking at people and seeing how the world kept going even in spite of my desperation, how it all seemed to go on as usual, how nobody noticed.

At some point around 46th Street I stopped dead on my tracks and in the midst of the bustle that is New York City I looked up at the sky and clearly stated out loud:

"Dear God, this is a bit much for me. I will keep on putting one foot in front of the other but You take care of the big details cause this is frigging out of my range"

And then I did put one foot in front of the other, one breath following the previous breath, one moment following the other. I continued living.

Looking back I can say that many things contributed to get me through the storm and bring me back to a place of balance, happiness, stability and even reinvention. These are 16 of them:

1. Kept up the yoga practice, every day.

2. Realized that I wanted to be happy rather than right, meaning that I worked at controlling any tendency of my mind to take me into a hole of depression.

3. Gave away 90% of my possessions -kind of had no choice, I was selling the house-. Ended up being the best decision of my life.

4. Allowed myself the opportunity to cry and feel like a failure. Then washed my face and kept going, one breath at the time.

5. Remained friends with the Human Resources person, I like her. Even in the midst of my fears I could tell that she was also trying to do her best within very difficult circumstances.

6. Volunteered for NYCares, surprisingly that was one of the most rewarding and healing things I did. Helping others ended up helping me. Funny, I know.

7. Woke up every morning to coffee, shower, and getting dressed. I meant business regardless of what the so-called "reality" suggested.

8. Started dating again and kept actively and purposely socializing.

9. Chanted the Gayatri mantra which I had just learned in Thailand—see resources- and like I meant it.

10. Cooked and ate at home all the time. Learned a few dishes by the way, I can make a mean curry.

11. Did not just look for jobs but after interviews I wrote lists to the potential employees with ideas of how they could improve their working situations (from the perspective of an IT Training Manager, which is what I was). I gave the ideas away without expectations. I came from a position of abundance, even though things around me could have suggested otherwise, I had

trust in the process, and I am not even sure where the strength came from, perhaps from having been practicing yoga for a while.

12. Talked to everyone under the sun, financial advisors, bankers, psychologists, wise women of my tribe, friends, friends of friends.

13. Did not waste energy on hating or blaming. Could not afford to.

14. Walked up every morning listing all the things I was grateful for (yoga, friends, love, my family in Argentina)

15. Meditated daily

16. Slept and ate as healthy as I could on my budget

Eventually, 6 months later, the house was sold without having to foreclose or short sell, taking a bit of a loss which was financed by borrowing from the 401K. The last mortgage payment was made with my last severance check. Somehow it all worked out.

I am eternally grateful for the lessons learned, and although I rather never have to go through it again, at least I know I survived by coming from a position of center and abundance.

The day after I was fired, on my next yoga class, when I told John Campbell (my then yoga teacher in New York

City) what had happened he said to me: "*This is your work now*". He meant yoga. I smiled.

How I Lost 30 Pounds Through Yoga And Never Saw them Again

Early in 2008 I set off for a trip to India. When I returned, I was 30 pounds lighter. The weight never came back.

A friend who knew me before the trip and then after it recently asked me how did this happen. As I tried to recall I noticed that it was not just because of the yoga, or the trip, or the food, or because I starved myself, and certainly not because I was mean or deprecating to myself in an attempt to discipline my food choices. None of that had anything to do with it.

Releasing weight can be a drama or not, it can be hard or not—it depends on so many factors that I do not believe one single method can ever work for everyone.

But these steps worked for me:

1-Loving Myself

There is no way around it, no matter who says that the US has an epidemic of whatever it might, or that I, or you, may need a diet or, that statistics show or blah, blah, blah, it is all nonsense if we do not start at the beginning. Loving and respecting me enough to sit down and look at what was important in life was the very first step.

I know it may sound silly but I followed Louise Hay's exercise of looking at myself in the mirror and saying "I love you", to my own image. At first it felt silly, stupid even, and you know why? Because I did not believe it. But a few weeks into it I did start to believe that I was worth of my own respect, and it helped me get grounded in acting as if I loved myself until I did eventually fully believe in it.

2-Daily Yoga-Asana Practice

I find that the release of the weight for me had to do with momentum rather than a get-thin-quick mentality. By the time I took my trip I had been practicing daily the yoga-asanas of primary series and for a year.

When it comes to releasing weight I find that it does not so much matter what kind of yoga one practices, but that one does. The simple act of getting on the mat every day sends the body the message that one cares. The body gets to be stretched, paid attention to, aligned.

With time my body began to take over, for example: it knew that we (body and mind) would have to enter kurmasana (tortoise pose) the following morning, and it knew that an empty stomach would make such exertions more palatable, and so it signaled me not to eat anything past 7 PM, a practice that has become a habit, because my body says so.

3-Verbal Messages

I find that people dismiss this quickly, so much so that I began to suspect it is a well-kept secret.

When somebody wants to manifest something positive, like achieving a healthy weight, then keeping the vocabulary clean (no curse words, no negativity) is key. It surprises me to no end to see, even in yoga circles, a tremendous denial of the power of the word. I hear people complain all the time, say bad/dirty/loaded words, and talk about their bodies with negativity.

Even as you read this, I will dare bet that you will either read through or dismiss it promptly. If you are still reading you are probably ready to hear it. If you are, then do not allow negativity into you, in any form. This in turn has the effect of cleansing the mind and to release bad ideas, extra anger and extra weight. Think of a diet of words as a foundation, the bad ones are very high in bad fats and calories.

There is a reason why I call it "weight release" (except perhaps in the title of this post), and that is because phrasing it that way is more powerful since usually whenever we lose something we try to find it again.

4- Cleansings

Weight release can also be thought of as cleansing. What is necessary is to look at what is coming into our bodies and how fast it is coming out. If we are not going to the bathroom (both for number one and two) daily, then there is a problem.

Just as an example, there are easy-to-use enema bags that help ensure that the internal pipes are clear. When I talk to friends about enemas they usually freak out, and so did I when I first heard about them. However I was blessed to have a teacher go over all of my fears and answer each one of them. Will it hurt? No, it does not. Will it be uncomfortable? Maybe but you are totally in control and can regulate the intensity.

Some people go all out and do a colonics treatment. Movie stars do these frequently because of the glow it produces. I have not tried one yet, but I want to. They are not too expensive and have an even deeper effect. And hey! If they are good for movie stars they are good for me too.

5-When Hungry, Drink Water First

A yoga teacher once said that to me. Most of us get the signal of hunger when in reality it is thirst speaking. I know I confuse the signals sometimes.

I have tried this many times, especially at mid-morning when I hear the stomach rumble with noise in what seems like starvation, and found that drinking one or two full glasses of water may not stop the feeling of wanting to eat, but at least will delay it. It will also hydrate the body, and help it with the elimination process.

6-Cooking

While in India I felt a little scared about eating in restaurants because the quality of their water is very dangerous for westerners so, for example, eating salads (or anything raw) outside of the house was not an option. This forced me to start cooking, and I prepared lots of stews and soups with boiled vegetables and olive oil which I served with brown rice.

Also I understood that very often our bodies are starving for real nutrition. For example, I learned that taking spirulina supplements is a great way of supplementing the diet so as not to have to eat a pound of spinach every day, or that Niacin (a type of B vitamin) helps enormously in uplifting moods. Of course this does not constitute medical advice, it is just what worked for me.

My constant investigations continue on even to this day. I am always looking for the best nutrition I can find for my body in particular. Lately for example I have noticed that flours are not so conducive to health for me, they tend to constipate the system, and so I try to avoid cupcakes, crackers and bread in general.

What is necessary is that each of us find what nurtures us, within this body, no point in forcing things or trying to copy what others do, just finding balance on what works for our own specific body. Yogis are personal laboratories of health and peace after all, whatever works is what we do.

7-Taking Time Off

Taking time for ourselves seems impossible, but it is not. When a body is overweight, it is out of balance. When a body is out of balance it needs time for itself, to heal, to have an opportunity to assess what exactly is happening and what can be done to help it. As long as the time we give to ourselves is dedicated, focused time, it is useful, otherwise we are not nurturing our soul, and an un-nurtured soul produces an unbalance that usually manifests in us reaching for the ice cream.

I have noticed that people who say that there is absolutely no way they can take time for themselves are actually saying that their priorities do not involve taking time off, meaning, their focus is not on their own wellbeing but rather on other things.

8-Surrendering

Our bodies are determined by our genes and ancestors. It is important to respect nature. Yoga and these principles can restore our body to our original blue-print, to what our bodies would be like if completely healthy, but they will not transform us into super models. The real miracle in weight release happens when we shift perception, when we can accept our body as it is and treat it well, with respect, providing good nutrition for it, so that it can function at its peak, which also means, mind you, at its ideal weight.

9.-Choosing The Middle Path

Trying to eat only spinach, or only drink water with lemon for days and nothing else, or going completely raw overnight or any other extreme is not only unrealistic, it is also dangerous and guaranteed to never work because we are fighting against a very powerful force of nature: our own natural psychological tendencies, which have been ingrained into us over a period of well, think about your age, that long.

In yoga this has to do with our *gunas* or psychological tendencies, of which there are three, rajasic or overexcited, tamasic or lethargic and satvic or balanced.

Forcing ourselves on being always balanced is in itself like forcing, because we are trying to machete our way through into the middle path rather than respecting what is actually happening right now. When we resist what is we fall unconscious. Falling into denial by trying to force a balanced energy is not the answer.

For example, a few months ago I felt like eating marshmallows. These are not exactly healthy treats as they have gelatin and are full of sugar, but I was fortunate enough at that very moment to be listening to Richard Freeman's *Yoga Matrix* and to hear exactly the message of this point, and so I ended up enjoying the marshmallows, going along with my tendencies, which was, albeit counterintuitive, the most satvic or balanced thing I could have done. I just observed what was happening but did not try to make it right. Interestingly, I have not felt the urge to eat them again, ever since.

10.- Trusting Our Instincts

Before every meal ask: what is the most nutritious thing I can eat right now? and trust, and let your body have it. Remember moderation, of course, but do go ahead. It may be decadent chocolate mud pie today, it might be baby spinach salad with fresh olive oil sprinkled with raw almonds tomorrow.

One thing I have found helpful recently is to stick to a plan for the week and have one cheat day in which I can eat anything I want, within reason. Even in spite of the within reason warning, in the beginning I was eating like crazy on that cheat day, but the interesting thing is that after a few weeks of noticing how the cheat day affected my week in general I began to be more mindful even in those days in which I could go all out.

11- Twelve Step Meetings

There is a cathartic effect in admitting our vulnerability to other people, as for instance when someone confesses to a group of people that he or she ate two pints of ice-cream the night before, or when someone says: "I am powerless over this". 12 step meetings work because they are simple steps that demand enormous courage, of the type that can only be navigated with help from others who also happen to find themselves in a similar setting.

The benefit of 12 steps meetings is that they open people up, they reconcile people with their own humanity, through them we find that what we think is crazy in us, is just as normal as it is in any other person, we all share a common humanity, we are all one, and I have yet to see a form of therapy that is more effective than people being brutally honest in a group, and under very specific regulations for sharing, with proper boundaries and respect.

12- Patience

Recovering a healthy body may take time, but every day things speed up, there is a momentum that is generated by slowly adding more and more healthy habits and releasing the old ones that do not serve us anymore.

A Yogi's Guide to Finding the Man Or Woman Of Your Dreams

Love does not hurt, it feels really good.
Oprah Winfrey

Sexual energy is the most powerful energy human beings have been bestowed with, yet its power confuses us and leaves us in a blur. Finding a life partner within the confines of a committed relationships is a vital step for a yogi so that the sexual energy can be properly channeled towards a person we trust and love.

Some people prefer to travel solo and that is a valid choice but in my experience I have seen that most people prefer to be in a relationship. At least in my case this was always what I wanted, only thing was that finding the right match was not an easy quest.

The important part is to always remember that we need to love ourselves first, and become the energy of the person we want to attract. We need to model the type of life we want to share, and a solid relationship starts with the one we have with ourselves.

Everyone is different but these steps offer guideposts against which at least we can test if we are being honest with ourselves. It is critical to find truth within us and notice if what we want is to play games and flirt and create intrigue, or if we really want a committed serious relationship. There is a world of difference between the two.

Having been in both extremes I can say that a real relationship based on love and honestly brings a lot of energy into the table, and allows each member of the couple to be their best, to grow, to expand.

1.-Brahmacharya: Well-Directed Sexual Energy

The first yoga principle relating to our modern times issue of dating and relationships is *brahmacharya*. It is listed in the Yoga Sutras, Chapter 2, sutra 38: *Upon establishment of celibacy, power is attained.*

Brahmacharya means celibacy, however common wisdom as well as endless interpretations from teachers of all times point to the understanding that what is meant for it is that we **use our sexual energy efficiently**. After all, even Krishnamacharya's teacher –whose name was Brahmachari- told him to go out into the world, build a family and teach yoga.

So, what does this mean for us? It means that when we find a partner we make a commitment to just have sexual relations with him or her, but also, to be truthful even before then, while on the search for a partner.

It means that we do not stay with someone we are dating just because of perceived personal gain, or that after seeing red-alert kinds of signals, or because of money, status, or anything else other than because real trust, support, and the possibility of love is present.

2.-Efficiency of Resources

Sexual energy is our vital force, a yogi recognizes this and uses it for the purpose of advancing on the spiritual path. This does not mean it gets to be secluded in a cave, on the contrary, yogis are encouraged to live in the world and have homes.

Like Marianne Williamson says: *We don't enter the kingdom of heaven alone, we go in pairs.*

It is through relationships that we learn the biggest and most important lessons in life. Only by having a close mirror, a direct feedback system that can identify our blind spots, our areas that need growth and change. And so, searching for a couple to share life with is important for a yogi.

3.-Getting Clear

Example: "I want a man/woman that has a good heart, does yoga, can speak Italian, is taller than me, loves to talk about spirit and do yoga, is ambitious, a good listener, always speaks the truth, loves me for exactly who I am, is generous and enjoys travel and popcorn during movies. I want a solid real relationship, based on truth and love, based on both of us wanting the other to grow, and to be happy".

Go ahead, write your own version, do write it down, and get SPECIFIC. Many people discard this step and file it under the category of "stupid" or "restrictive". Big mistake, consider Alice story's moral:

One day Alice came to a fork in the road and saw a Cheshire cat in a tree. Which road do I take? she asked. Where do you want to go? was his response. I don't know, Alice answered. Then, said the cat, it doesn't matter

Many people say they want a relationship, but by not being clear they perhaps fail to notice that what they really want is actually drama, they feel invisible and so they create complicated situations with unavailable people so that they sound interesting. Becoming aware of this behavior is a first step, clarifying what we really want would be the next.

4.-Intend, Detach, Trust

A Yogi recognizes the power of the word, the power of intention, the power of being clear about what it is one wants. That is what step 3 is for, to set the intention, to make it clear.

Once the intention is clear it is important to release it so that the universe can fold itself in magical ways and act as catalyst to attract exactly that which you say you want, provided of course, you are detached and open to all possibilities. It may not be 100% what you wrote, but I find you may be surprised. We never know exactly how things will happen, nobody does, and that is not up to you or me, that is up to destiny. Once we are clear we can work at being present, at giving our full attention to whatever situation comes our way, rooted in trust that the universe is sending the right circumstances.

5.-Clean Vocabulary

When somebody wants to manifest a new and healthy relationship in their lives keeping the vocabulary clean is vital.

Not only that but also if you keep saying "Oh I am too old nobody will ever want me", then that is what you are putting out and that is what you will get.

Train yourself to say things like "I am open to the right man or woman to come into my life" "There is an abundance of men and the right one is attracted to me"

Forget naysayers. They are in the majority and they have not read this book yet. That is OK, maybe they are not ready to hear it, maybe they prefer drama, bless them and continue on your path to finding love.

Note that I am not advocating denial, sometimes things are difficult. Keeping it real is also important, the key is to find the right balance.

6.-Body, Mind, Spirit

To attract the coolest man in the world the best recipe is to become the coolest woman in the world. I first heard those words from a Marianne Williamson CD, and it resonated deeply.

Do you feel good? Are you eating healthy? Are you practicing your yoga? How about your clothes? Do you reflect the happy person you want to be? Is your hair tidy? Is your home tidy?

Ensuring that body mind and spirit are working together is important, you need to have a good foundation and become what you want to attract. If you would like a generous sexy partner, start by becoming that yourself. Take care of you first.

7.-Socializing In The Right Places

I am surprised when I hear men ask where can they meet women. Easy! yoga classes, tango classes, painting classes, cooking classes.

As per women, there are plenty of places too: salsa classes, tango classes, chess clubs, meetups.

Thinking that there are no men or that there are no women is not true. It is just a sentence that our mind likes to throw into the mix to keep us small. There are plenty of good men looking for food women and the same applies the other way around. It is important to keep the social life active, to take that salsa class, go to that tango or zumba class. Or go to a Meetup that enjoys going to museums, or talking sustainability. Try everything that aligns with things you like. Get out there and mingle.

Dating sites can work too, they worked for me! But for dating sites to be effective all other steps must be very much in place, and this is because of the nature of the introductions (i.e.: both parties come in expecting a date and with certain preconceptions/expectations).

8.-The One Hour Cup Of Tea

When I was dating I had a one hour cup of tea rule for people I met for the first time. This was convenient because it allowed me enough time to share a conversation with no strings attached (i.e.: nobody had to pay for an expensive dinner) and most importantly, it came with a clear exit strategy for me. If it did not work out, then one hour was not a long time and nobody's feelings got hurt. If it did work out it provided a safe container in which to talk and make plans for a future date.

Through this method I met many men over coffee, tea, hot chocolate and, once, bubble tea. Whenever they offered to go for dinner I kindly declined, even if I liked them. This gave me the buffer of time of another date, a little time to settle in, check with my spirit, see how I felt, see if I had changed my behavior to try to please, see if I was going overboard, exaggerating things, see if the person I became when in front of him was really myself or if I was acting out some kind of a fantasy me (not a good sign).

9.- No Bed For 13 Dates

The bed part of a relationship must be handled with care. It is important to get to know the person before the sexual communication begins, otherwise sex tends to color things, make it all strange, a little awkward, and you know what? The right man will wait, if he does not want to, then he is simply not the right man. Read that again, it was the best advise my friend Michele ever gave me.

Many women feel they need to get in bed to hold on to a man (I know because when I was younger I felt that way), this reflects a huge insecurity, a thinking that perhaps we are not interesting enough and so we have to take our clothes off to keep things alive. The reality is that what is more intimate and sexy is to open up slowly, to let him discover you, to share stories, laugher, walks, to really get to know the other person, to become best friends. The sex part will take care of itself.

As a guideline, try to stay away from bed for at least 13 dates. And yes, I know that many people will disagree with this. Is the number arbitrary? Yes it is, absolutely, it is what worked for me, perhaps you can make up your own, just make sure it works and that you are not sabotaging yourself.

10.-Community Support

I did not learn how to handle relationships until I was in my late 30s. All the insecurities I described above I had. All of them, no exceptions.

I cried so many times over perceived broken hearts and unavailable men, that one day I decided I wanted to learn what I was doing wrong. To begin with I attended meetings at the SLAA, (Sex and Love Addicts Anonymous).

I realized that I had an "addiction to love" because I always ended up not just in love with someone but obsessed and always with men that were not available. If a man was interested in me then I enjoyed playing hard to get. I was into intrigue and drama, and not putting the energy where it would better serve a relationship.

Love addiction is one of those things nobody likes to talk about, it is sticky, embarrassing, and often shuffled under the rug. In those rooms, which are free and anonymous, you hear deep conversations that nobody shares over a drink, or at home, or in the office. So much so that I think sex is a bigger taboo than money. We are afraid of speaking the truth of it. Not only that, but also love addiction has another side to it which is sexual anorexia, a condition by which some people feel compelled to stay at home and not go anywhere, ever. Sexual anorexia is exactly that, a starvation of our soul in the area of relationships. Might be worth going to one meeting just to listen in and see if anything resonates.

The important thing about these meetings for me is that I built a community of support through them. When I was dating I had 10 people I could call at any given time to run a reality check, see if I was rushing into things, if I was trying to please, if I was forgetting about what I really wanted, if I was acting out. A great resource while navigating the deep waters of new relationships.

11.-Keeping The Life You Have

Ensure to keep your own life going when you are dating, do not stop going to yoga or doing the activities that bring you joy. Remember you will not be building a life together for a while, becoming two is transitional work, it takes time, and the slower and most awkward the better.

12.- It's Work!

You are on the search for the relationship of your life, for your soul partner, so it is a good idea to consider it a serious assignment. It is a good suggestion to schedule things and approach it seriously. To give it the energy it needs when it comes to getting clear and planning. Once we are clear and grounded we can work at staying present, at being who we are, and remaining open to the circumstances that the universe will present us. We can flow with life as it is. . It is true that it takes energy but the payoff is beautiful, rewarding, loving, and amazing.

SEVEN: 15 UNUSUAL BENEFITS OF YOGA

On a previous chapter I talked about the specific benefits of the primary series of Ashtanga yoga as described by Pattabhi Jois himself. In this chapter I would like to share with you the more practical, day-to-day benefits it has brought into my own life, those that come with the serious, steady, and dedicated daily practice.

As I write this line, seven years after Ashtanga yoga awoke my curiosity for the first time, my life has been thoroughly transformed for the better. I am doing work I love, practicing every day, learning the first poses of the intermediate series, living in a peaceful setting, and happy.

Through the practice I have been able to gather enough momentum and resources to travel to remote areas of the world and learn about new cultures and traditions. I have become clear about relationships and started channeling my energies towards the creative projects that resonate with my spirit. All in all, it has been really good to me. The following are some very specific benefits I reaped so far:

1.- Discipline

Ever since I came into Ashtanga, the word discipline took on a new and different meaning, a visceral one. Now I understand at a cellular level what it means to have a practice, and I like it.

I find that this has transcended into other areas of my life, I realize for example, that being present for conversations is also a practice, or minding the type of veggies I select when at the supermarket, or the way the spinach is washed, or how each word is pronounced as I learn to recite the Yoga Sutras in Sanskrit. A whole new level of awareness has come into my life through the practice of yoga as a discipline.

2.- Better Breathing

My husband used to joke with me when we were dating that I could tell when his breathing pattern changed and that nobody had pointed this out to him before.

Nowhere have the benefits been more clear than in the way I breathe. I now notice how the air flows in and out at every moment. I notice when it gets shorter, and when it's deep. Just the simple awareness has improved the quality of my life, I now know when I need to slow down, take a break, rest, or when I am slugging and procrastinating.

Yogis measure their longevity in breaths rather than in years, and when this shift happens in our conscious we begin to savor each one of them.

3.-Efficiency

Getting on the mat every day for an hour and a half or two has taught me to use my energy with care, to ensure it will last for the session. This again has repercussions as I go through the day, for example, I notice the way in which I am speaking. Am I using too much energy or speaking too loudly? Am I trying too hard where it is not necessary? Maybe trying to convince someone of something?

The constant questioning of my underlying intentions in each action brings presence to each situation and makes me more useful and grounded.

The deeper level awareness of my limited human energy has made it all the more relevant in life when off the mat, and I can also detect quickly where there are clogs, where the energy gets obstructed, for example: Do I own too many things that I do not need? Must I really buy an extra bed cover for the Spring season?, or would I just like it for a while and then not use it?

Questions like this appear every day, they built themselves into my stream of consciousness and help me direct my limited resources in a more productive way.

4.- I Stopped Complaining

I find that complaining is the biggest obstacle to success in any field. It is a waste of energy and a leak in the system. When I was into it, it was a great enabler for me to let the victim archetype show and take over. Never a good conduit for growth or creativity.

The main reason why complaining is a waste of energy is because the ego likes to tell us how we are special and separate from everything else, how our suffering justifies us getting lost in thought and avoiding being present, how fueling our discontent keeps the mind occupied and gives her a sense of existence.

Complaining goes against the yogic principle of contentment or Santosha, and it is another well kept yoga secret. If you try to stop complaining for a week, or even for a day you will see how difficult it can be. This shows how engrained the process is with our daily living. I have made a commitment to stop for a week and to start counting again whenever I find myself slipping. I have yet to see a whole week go by. That is why it is a practice.

5.- Dealing With Difficult Situations

Yoga did not make life easier, but it gave me a better set of choices and tools on how to deal with dramatic events.

Drama is something I try to avoid these days and although it is impossible to completely eradicate it, I realize that at least the cheap drama can be let go of.

But life is suffering, that is the first precept the Buddha (an enlightened being) taught, and he is right, being a yogi does not make anyone exempt from having stuff happening to them. It is the way in which we react that changes, the level of awareness with which we approach life's challenges.

6.- Purification

Yoga has had a profound cleaning effect in me. Practicing the primary series consistently and over time helped me become more regular in the processes of elimination and in my cycles. It also helped me rest better.

But the cleansing has gone a lot further. Now-a-days my house is also clean, as is the closet and the sheets in the bed. My books are in order and so are my finances. It is not perfect but it is a work in progress and the aim is for total transparency, one day at the time.

Cleansing is very connected to efficiency. It is about using all resources, including the ones in my body efficiently, it is as much as letting the internal pipes of my body flow as it is for having the dishwasher work without an overload of dishes.

7.- Curving Drama

Drama has abandoned me for the most part. Not completely but I find that the deeper I go into yoga and the more I learn about using energy in a resourceful way, the less drama there is in my life, or if there is, my reaction to it is not so intense.

There is a story called a second arrow which illustrates this beautiful. It suggests that if you were hit by an arrow you would be in pain, but if you were then hit by a second one you would be in even more pain. The punch line of the story is that the second arrow is your own reaction to the first one.

9.- Word Choices

I believe that the best kept secret in our world is the power of the word as I have mentioned. How we phrase things, the way in which we say what we want to say means the difference between a broken relationship and a flourishing one, between a success or a failure, between a gentle continuation or an abrupt stop in a practice. Words are powerful, they are spells we cast. Taking a moment to honor them, and to choose them with care brings about an abundance of new possibilities.

10.- Synchronicity

Synchronic events were there all along, I was just not noticing them. Since I started practicing I began finding answers in the most unusual places. In the plates of cars, in a giant wheel I saw on the way to the airport as I went to India (which I understood as a turning of the wheel in my life). There are so many examples of big coincidences that sometimes my life feels like a science fiction novel.

11.- Life As Dedication To The Divine

Letting all the results of our actions be up to that Higher Power that keeps us alive in this very moment is a lesson worth practicing.

Living as dedicating our lives to a higher purpose changes things, it makes us more aware, it shows each moment for what it is, sacred, and hence helps us being more rooted on what is rather than our mental projections and speculations of what we want it to be.

12.- Creativity

Yoga helps creativity soar, perhaps due to the more efficient use of resources I have found that room for wandering and creativity just happens and the results are very rewarding. For example: I have found an enormous community of friends and yogis through the creativity expressed in my blog and I find that writing has become a practice, a creative one, just like yoga.

13.- Scriptures

I have begun to learn new ideas directly from the scriptures, going deeper into the philosophy behind yoga. This happens sooner or later to any serious student of yoga, curiosity is natural and human. We get into the deeper layers, we find new meaning.

14.- Awe and Curiosity

Curiosity has been awakened, I am ever so interested in the journey in how the universe unfolds and rearranges to teach me, to nurture me. When you trust, everything is supporting you and your creativity, your work, your life.

15.- Peace

I have found peace, not all the time, not every moment, but at a deeper level I am fundamentally a much more peaceful person since yoga came into my life.

The question I always ask when presented with difficult situations is do I want this or do I want peace? The immediate answer tends to get me on the right track right away.

EIGHT: CASTOR OIL BATH: THE ASHTANGA YOGA SATURDAY PRACTICE

Saturdays are the days of rest in the Ashtanga tradition and I, for one, am very fond of them. I appreciate the opportunity to let my muscles relax and rest and the opportunity to have coffee and read without the mat deadline.

The first time I travelled to India I heard from many practitioners that they had been advised by Pattabhi Jois to do what is called the "Saturday Practice", by which they meant a castor oil bath.

The bath is said to be so powerful that common wisdom recommends taking it very easy on the following Sunday practice as the body is prone to be much more supple and stretching might seem easier, tempting one to go further than usual and increasing the chance for injury.

If you are thinking of trying it, it might be useful to talk to a teacher before attempting, just to be on the safe side.

The benefit of the bath is in the heat that the oil produces in the body. Every time I bathe in the oil I feel as if I had a suit on me that is trapping and then releasing impurities. Further benefits among others are the reduction of pain and inflammation and a healthy glow.

I usually get the Castor Oil that can be found in any health food store. Some readers of my blog have suggested that sesame or even almond oil can also be used.

I use one medium bottle per bath (about a pint). Then I follow these steps:

1.- Ensure that you have a surface covered either with a towel or some sort of floor protection. Things are about to get messy.

2.- Sit on the towel , pour oil on your head, and massage the scalp, then continue by pouring oil all over your body and gently massage it.

3.- Lay in corpse pose and relax for about 10 to 15 minutes. Best not to overdo it, especially the first time, as you are testing the effect that this practice will have on you.

4.- Carefully (as all surfaces you step on will be slippery if you rubbed your feet), step into the shower and remove the oil. I use a citrus soap, which works very well as it seems to cut the grease. Then shampoo one or two times and condition if you want to.

5.- Once you think you have taken all the oil out of your body, it may be a good idea to soap up again. The oil is very sticky and you probably have not taken it all out, I know because this happens to me every time.

6.- Clean the shower so the next person coming in does not slip and fall.

7.- Get dressed and take it easy. Just to give you an example, I am writing this post after taking the castor oil bath and I am feeling a mix of relaxation, a sense of wellbeing, and an urgent desire to lay down. As soon as I am done writing I will do just that. Be especially careful not to go under the sun afterwards, and if you live in an area with cold weather, dress warm and drink plenty of water.

8.- Finally, and perhaps most importantly be careful in your Sunday asana practice. Take it easy and never push beyond your edge.

NINE: WHEN THE TIME COMES: VISITING MYSORE, IN SOUTH INDIA

You may be curious after you start your practice about the Ashtanga Yoga Research Institute (AYRI) in Msyore, South India. Also, if you are lucky you may have Sharath, Saraswathi, or Manju come on tour to a city near you, and that is an experience not to be missed. After that, Mysore is really it.

The city is a place of wonder. People from India consider it the country-side, although I would disagree a little as my first impression of it was that of a very busy metropolis.

Coming to Mysore, specifically to the AYRI is a great treat to focus on your practice.

I find that it might be better to visit when your practice is not yet so advanced because you have less attachments to it. But any time is good and everyone is welcome. Just make sure to read on so you know the drill.

Tips for Safe Travels to India

Visiting India can be safe but precautions need to be taken because the sanitation standards are different.

Before I left for Mysore on my second trip I visited a doctor and got some advice, I also learned lots from my very own roommates in India, and collectively here is the knowledge I have gathered

1- Don't Let Tub Water Into Your Mouth

Water in India is unsafe, so when you are showering close your mouth and be especially careful when washing your hair.

Just to give you an example, one of my roommates did not believe this and one night brushed her teeth with tub water. She felt bad in the morning, skipped yoga practice and ended up staying in bed for two whole days. She had diarrhea and vomit spurs and got completely dehydrated.

You may be one of those people with a hard stomach that can handle anything, if so, then you are in luck, but if I was you, at least on the first trip, I would be cautious.

2- Don't Eat Raw Food That Has Been Sitting

At first try to stick to the touristy (read western oriented) restaurants, and do not eat lettuce or raw produce in restaurants because they wash them with the water you are avoiding. Eat at home instead when you feel like raw.

Also, when the weather is very hot, consider that some buffet restaurants leave the food out for long stretches of time and bacteria can get to them. This is not to scare you out of eating out, just to be careful on very hot days.

3- Take Water Purification Liquids With You

I add a few drops of Liquid Grapefruit seed oil to the water with which the vegetables will be washed.

When cooking at home I concentrated on stews. Beans are a plenty, at least in the Mysore area, and it is so cheap to cook at home that it seems like an exercise in living in an affordable world, very much so.

For all raw vegetables always make it a point to take all dirt out and if possible wash them twice.

5- Diarrhea / Vomiting

It might happen, even if you take all precautions. It is always good to be prepared for the worst case scenario so it is important to talk to the doctor and ask for an anti-diarrhea pill and to also ask for something to stop vomiting.

My doctor suggested that if it came to this point, to first let it run out before I started taking the anti-diarrhea stuff (Imodium). I know this might be a little too much information and I consider myself lucky that I did not get to that point ever. Should you encounter yourself there, it is good to know.

6- Take Re-Hydration Pills With You

But remember to drink plenty of filtered water. When one of my friends was sick due to poorly cleaned food I offered some of the re-hydration pills I had carried with me and she said she felt as a plant would after being close to dying and receiving some water. They can come quite handy, I found them in Amazon.

7 – Flash Light and Umbrella

Remember to pack them and carry them with you.

During the 2008 trip the power cuts were as frequent as unpredictable, and the streets were not paved. There are lots of holes everywhere so it is really handy to have a flash light. As per the umbrella, it will come handy if you visit during Monsoon season, at least until you get used to the timing of when the showers are likely to come by.

8- Mosquito Net

I brought my own which I borrowed from a friend who had gone to Africa. It was a cool thing to have and I could see how it could have come handy depending on where I would rent a space. I was lucky that my room in a big house near the AYRI did not need a net, but there were plenty of mosquitoes around.

9- Dress Appropriately If You Are A Woman

The customs of India are very different than in the West so it is a sign of respect to wear a shawl over your shoulders if you are a woman and in general to keep the dressing modest (no mini-skirts for example, no tight pants). As a good rule, anything that would call attention to you in your own country will probably double in India. Talk to other women and find out what is suitable.

I normally wear t-shirts with short sleeves that cover my shoulders in full and a shawl on top, and pants or long skirts. Sometimes I also wear a dress but never skip the shawl.

It may feel strange in the beginning but you may end up liking them and using them all the time, even when back home.

Men do not seem to have much of a problem with the dressing part, the only notorious thing perhaps is that Indian men seem to never wear shorts, but I never saw any man get in trouble by wearing them.

My Packing List for Each Visit

Maybe the most important thing on my packing list were ear-plugs, as people in Mysore seem to drive with their hands attached to the horn and they will blow it constantly.

I have a feeling they get a secret pleasure out if, as if the sound would provide proof of existence: they make loud noises therefore they exist. Not a bad way to protect the ego, I suppose, especially in a country where so many Gods are looking at you from every angle.

This is packing list that I compiled throughout the years, you may not need every single item in it but having it on the list at least gives you the possibility of considering it before you board.

YOGA BOOKS for inspiration –see resources-. Especially if you are going for a long stretch of time (8 weeks or longer), you may crave your own books. There are places where to buy books in English there, for example Rashinkar (the tailor) has some near the shala and a huge variety in his shop downtown, or the Ramakrishna ashram. However, I always like to bring my own inspiration, and in the days of the kindle things are a lot easier.

MOSQUITO REPELLENT. You can find this in stores in India but I prefer to bring the one I am used to.

MOSQUITO NET. for the bed. Not completely necessary but a nice to have, just in case.

IMODIUM or other over thecounter medication for possible diarrhea.

NAUSEA PREVENTING PILLS. Always good to be prepared.

PROBIOTICS. This may apply only to me or not, thing is, if you take them at home it is good to have them on the list to remember as finding them in Mysore may prove difficult.

YOGA PRACTICE CLOTHES. Remember that it is pretty hot in Mysore, especially between February and June.

YOGA MAT. There are stores now-a-days that sell them there, but I find I like to have my own mat, besides it is best for the environment to just have one mat.

MYSORE RUG. The Mysore rug is a cloth rug that is usually placed on top of the regular mat to absorb sweat. I bought my latest Mysore rug at the AYRI because I liked the ones they had and they seemed to stick and give better traction. You can get them at the shop within the shala which usually opens every day in the afternoons.

YOGA WATER SPRAYER (in case you need to wet your legs before rolling around in *garbha pindasana*)

LITTLE TOWELS for practice. You can buy them a plenty on the main road in Gokulam itself, but if you have a preference it is good to have them on the list.

TEA TREE OIL. Useful to mix with water and spray the mat, so that it gets clean

PASSPORT, PHOTOCOPIES, EXTRA PHOTOS. You will need to provide a copy of your passport when you register at the shala and possibly to your landlord, and maybe even if you want to buy a phone or a sim card, so get a few of those in your bag. As per passport pictures it is a good idea to bring with you at least 2, you never know when you may need one.

HYDRATION PILLS

ELECTRICITY PLUG CONVERTERS

LAPTOP. Internet connectivity is one of the good news about Mysore. It is a lot easier to get connected these days. I bought an adaptor that came with broadband and could be connected to any USB entry port in the notebook

PHONE that hopefully will work there. It might be good to do research on this depending on what phone you have. Also find out about plans and costs to avoid surprises upon return.

SANDALS or easy shoes

SUN PROTECTOR

SWIMMING SUIT. There are a few pools in the area if you are into it, see the guide to Mysore in a future chapter.

EAR PLUGS

EYE MASK

PRESENTS for the people of the house where you might be staying –usually sweet butter cookies will do-

NETI POT AND SALT. If you walk around or take a trip to downtown Mysore you will find that the air can get very polluted. It is good to run salty water through the nostrils –as in the practice of using a neti pot- to keep the breathing organs clean.

GRAPEFRUIT OIL to put in the water that will wash vegetables

FLASHLIGHT. I prefer to bring one from home so I don't have to buy a big one there.

CAMERA. You will want to record your memories, although nowadays phones seem to come with cameras that even record video, we are lucky to live in these times.

UMBRELLA. Very important during monsoon season.

CALL THE BANK before you go so that they do not stop you from withdrawing all the rupees you will need to take out.

TEN: AN ASHTANGA YOGA GUIDE TO MYSORE, INDIA

I have been to Mysore a few times and I always felt that it would be good to have a comprehensive guide that would tell me where to buy the essential things you are sure to need and also those exotic things you may want to check out. I wanted a guide like that so much that I went ahead and created one. To see it you can visit www.mysorepedia.com that is Mysore Pedia Dot Com, I bought the domain so it would be easy to remember.

Throughout the years the list grew as other fellow students and friends shared with me places that they have visited and they liked.

I keep on updating the list all the time. You will see that it is a bit "mom-and-pops", but it can help you in those first couple of days until you get your bearings.

Not all the places I list have their own websites yet, so it is best to visit mysorepedia.com for up to date info, links to photos, etc.

However I found that having the list in print helped me one time when I had just arrived and did not have internet yet, so here it comes. As usual, checking online will give you more up to date information. You know the drill.

Yoga

<u>Ashtanga Yoga Research Institute</u>. Make sure to register early through their website kpjayi.org, as it fills up quickly. When you arrive and are ready to register bring a passport picture and photocopy of your passport page and visa page. Registration is usually done in the afternoons, between 3:30 and 4:30 but make sure to ask around as things can change.

One good thing to know about the Institute, at least as of 2011, is that it has what is called: "shala time", which is different than real time and by 15 minutes. So always think that they are 15 minutes ahead, and for whatever time they tell you get there early. See this <u>article</u> for the story behind the shala time:
<u>http://earthyogi.blogspot.com/2011/01/dealing-with-greed-love-doubt.html</u>

Accommodations

Many students just walk around Gokulam and knock on doors. Indian families are opening their doors to students more and more, and this is the most inexpensive way to find a room as well as get a real experience of how a family in Southern India lives. In my experience I have found them to be very friendly and hospitable people.

In later years the prices have been raising however, perhaps due to the enormous demand that the institute puts on living in the area near its doors. Planning in advance is a good thing if you can do it.

As a reminder, for further linking and photographs visit mysorepedia.com

The Green Hotel is a beautiful and soft landing for the first couple of nights. A bit pricey, but worth the night. They also serve fine food. http://www.greenhotelindia.com/

Anokhi Garden **Bed and Breakfast** - They have a few rooms and a beautiful studio, again, must reserve early. http://www.anokhigarden.com/

Hotel Metropole. Have not seen it yet, but I have heard good things about their food. Apparently it is a bit high-end, mostly for business people, so it might be a bit more pricey, but nice. It is a Rickshaw drive from the shala.

Hotel Paradise. My friends were staying in this hotel for the first couple of nights so I got to see it. I was not crazy about the food, but the hotel seemed to have a lot of room.

Transportation

Right by the shala there is a Rickshaw stand where you can find Seddu, one of the nicest and lively drivers around, he can take you to any of the places listed here. Ph 9880417398. In general a short drive (say from the shala to the supermarket: Loyal World) would cost about 30 rupees, maybe 40 as of 2012, prices are likely to vary of course depending on when you go.

Wait time is about 25 to 50 rupees per hour if you want a driver to wait for you while you shop. Seddu is of course not the only driver, and he can recommend others that can help. They are all very respectful and will pick you up on time.

Krishna arranged **car rides** from Bangalore Airport in great cars, with seat belts and all (was not the case in 2008). E-mail: tskittymurthy@yahoo.co.in - Price is about 50 dollars each way. If you get to go in a group, make sure to pay 50 for the group, not for each person.

Food and Internet

Dosalicious. Mint dosas? Fusion Dosa? Fusion Idly? Yes!, I know, I am also having trouble believing but it is true.

Santosha, is about two blocks from the shala and serves brunch every day 8-12, closed on Saturdays. They seem to change owners every two or three years, but the place seems to be blessed with a permanent friendly atmosphere and good food. Santoshamysore.com

Sri Durga, or the "Stand Up Cafe", Indian breakfast and lunch. The food comes out quickly and pretty much everything is tasty, the prices are very cheap, as in a full meal could be about 16 rupees.

Anokhi Garden Bed and breakfast, has brunch every day except Monday and Tuesday. On Saturdays it gets very crowded as many other places are closed so go early, other than that the food is very tasty. Anokhigarden.com

Vivian's Cafe, open for brunch every day except Saturday, they are on the same street as the shala, so it is nice to just stroll in after practice. Their French toasts are small but their fruit salads are huge (as of 2012). Wireless is available.

Tina's Cafe is a favorite for many students, and is open 1 to 1 PM every day except Sundays.

The Austrian Cafe, a bit of a walk as it is not precisely in Gokulam, they have burgers, chicken and tiramisu... certainly different. You can find them near Loyal World (the supermarket).

Chakra House. The last day of my second trip to Mysore I had had brunch with a full plate of eggs veggie, potatoes, chai and juice for 110 ruppias... and the best news is that they are open for breakfast, lunch, AND dinner, EVERY DAY. If you like to drink your chai with your breakfast order it "right away", otherwise they think chai is kind of like a dessert, other than that, enjoy the food, it is nice. As of 2012 they were on the yellow house near the shala.

Authana Restaurant. Great dosas and Indian food in general, they follow the schedule of Indian restaurants where dinner is served at around 7 but during the day they have "snacks" which usually means Chinese noodles and dosa. They deliver!

Ganesh Internet and Cafe, is a great spot, close to the shala, and serves lunch at 1 and dinner at 5. It is a buffet and Anu (who is a great cook) prepares fresh meals. It is a great way to get your veggies in. The seating area for food is upstairs and they have wireless if you would like to bring your laptop. Students tend to Skype family from it and you will likely find people with headsets, eating great food and relaxing.

Green Leaf is an Indian Restaurant located about 15 minutes' walk from the Coconut stand. We went at "snack" time, and so we only got Chinese noodles and dosa but they have a very full menu for lunch and dinner. Seems to have a reputation for being noisy, but the food was very good.

Rishi's Cafe is run by a group of Indian women. You can come in and they will serve you food between 1 and 7 every day, except Sundays. They have amazing shakes. They also have computers and wireless.

The Chai place on Main Street: Amruth... is a must try! It could be a little intimidating as it is always filled with men, but fear not, women are welcome, and you will love it. Me thinks I may be a bit addicted to it. Try not to drink it too late (not past 4:00 PM) as it might be hard to go to sleep afterwards and you may be tempted to snooze that early alarm clock.

The Gokul Chats has huge and amazing dosa until 11 AM and from 5 PM. Not to be missed, it is the real Mysore food experience, and delicious

Sixth Main. I have eaten lunch here once and really liked it, but they pretty much respect the 1-2:30 or so lunch and 6 to 7 or so dinner. They are near the Loyal World supermarket. They deliver.

The internationally famous COCONUT STAND. This is it. Get your electrolytes for 10 rupees. You will find it right away as lots of students gather there in spite of Sharath telling us in many conferences to stay away from it and keep our energy to ourselves. Oh well, c'est la vie.

Barista, the Starbucks of Mysore, where you can find Indian locals smoking and playing chess, order a latte and have some sandwiches. It also has wireless but it seems to be inconsistent in service. It is also across the street from a major bank in case you need to withdraw some money, you can have a coffee and bank.

RRR. In downtown, an all amazing Indian experience, it is likely you will be the only foreigner there and the food is served without you having to ask for anything. Just get bottled water.

Pascucci – An Italian coffee-shop, it has a variety of coffee, sandwiches and salads, they also have wi-fi.
Pascucci.in

Hotel Mylari. Seddu took us to this place and I have to tell you it is an experience. The dosas are fluffy (thicker) and fried in butter, delish!

The Three Sisters. This is a place downtown where you need to call ahead and they will cook for you. I enjoyed a meal at their place in 2008 and loved it. They also offer ayurvedic massages! I heard that a book of their recipes has been compiled and published too.

Supermarkets

Loyal World, a five minute ride in a Rickshaw, they have everything from electronics to food.

More. Used to be called "Fab City", but now has a new name, it is near the market. The place is huge, akin to the "Target" or "Tesco" of Mysore. Whatever you may need, is there, except for ear-plugs which cannot be found anywhere in India that I know of.

Nilgris. This is the supermarket of Gokulam, relatively small, but pretty solid. They are on the main road, can't miss them.

The Coffee and Chocolate man. He and his wife run a tiny little shop near the shala and they really try to have everything. I try to go to them as often as I can. Their coffee is grind-ed in front of your eyes.

The Ayurvedic Oil Man

When I was here in 2008 a friend asked Guruji for some good oils to alleviate pain, and he sent him straight to this store. I have used his products and enjoyed them very much. He is used to students coming from the shala and will probably give you a mix of two oils to put before showering. The shop is located a few blocks from the shala next to the Gokul Chats (see food).

Tailors, Arts and Crafts

Rashinkar - I usually visit them downtown and get tailored dresses with Indian fabrics. They ship worldwide: rashinkar.com.

Krishna Tailor. He is in Gokulam close to the shala and has pre-made pants and shirts. He can also make things on demand.

The Heritage - This is a house of crafts, they have amazing fabrics, jewelry, statues, carpets and more. They ship world wide. theheritage2009@hotmail.com

Museum - Also a place of amazing quality fabrics, near the market.

Kauvery Silk Arts and Crafts. They tell me that all the artisans working here are representing the goverment of India which supposedly means good value and great work. See for yourself, some of the art work was indeed breath taking.

Bookstores

The Ramakrishna Ashram and Bookstore. Amazing place, a must see, and they are right in Gokulam.

Sapna, means "dream" and is perhaps the most "flashy" bookstore, a dream come true. They have 3 floors. I love their stationary island on the first floor and the amazing variety of mystic and craft books. The third floor is filled with text books. Very interesting. This is their website: http://www.sapnaonline.com/.

Rashinkar. Yes they are the tailors but they also have a good selection of books both downtown and in the Rashinkar "Mansion" across the street from the Mysore Lion's school in Gokulam.

Ashok Books. A somewhat smaller bookshop recommended for spiritual texts in English. It is actually quite close to Sapna.

Dentist

We found a great dentist, her name is Judith Pereira, and she is right next to Ganesh (see food). She was really nice, and offered very cheap services, for example, a root canal is 400 rupees. I know! Amazing! - She was trained in Germany and has a daughter in the US so she is familiar with the westerner culture.

Chanting

The shala has chanting and yoga sutra classes with Lakshimish. You need to inquire for details.

There is also of course the Anantha Research Foundation, where the famous Dr. M.A. Narasimhan and M.A. Jayashree can be found teaching yoga sutra classes.

Sightseeing

The Mysore Palace lights up every Sunday night, make sure to be there a few minutes before 7 PM, then get to sleep for practice! :-)

Wineye Vinay is a shala student and also a tour guide in Mysore, this is his website. He can take you to the Mysore that is local, hidden. He will make you step off beaten path... and he is a yogi, how cool is that?
http://www.royalmysorewalks.com/

Chamundi Hill is a must see which I have not seen yet! I hear it is a must. A You Tube video/documentary has been recently produced about the Swami that lives on the hill, Google it and you will see.

Jewlery

Silver Nest is the house of Meena, a sweet Indian woman who makes incredible silver necklesses, toe rings and pendants with the shape of the Indian Gods. Did I mention they are one block from the shala? Silvernest.net

Swiming Pool

The Regaalis Hotel used to be called "Souther Star" and is one of the swiming pools around. Make sure to go by before 5PM as, who knows why the arquitect did not think of this, but after 5 the sun is blocked by the building of the hotel! Anyway, they have great food and amazing cakes. The swimming pool is lovely and you will see lots of yogis striking a pose or two.

Lalhita Mahal Palace - the second largest palace in Mysore, also offers a swimming pool. It is a bit of a drive, not as close as the hotel above (from the point of view of Gokulam) but worth the visit.

Reporting Abuse

A few of us have been molested (slightly) while in Gokulam, if you happen to experience this, God protect you!, then grab the license plate of the motorcycle or yell so that people further down the street can catch the guy, then dial the number 100 from any indian phone (borrow someone's cell phone is free), and report it to the police.

A Final Word

Keep on visiting Mysore Pedia Dot Com for more up to date news, and more importantly, if you find a good place make sure to email and let me know at the blog or in Twitter (Twitter.com/ClaudiaYoga) and I will add it so we can all benefit, I will, of course, also give you credit.

ELEVEN: ADVENTURES OF A BEGINNER IN MYSORE

Coming to Mysore as a beginner is a test of vulnerability, endurance and strength. It is also a lot of fun. My husband took his first trip when he had only been practicing for six months and 3 times a week on average. This is the recount of his experience in Mysore after his second class:

Yoga has Completely Humiliated Me:

I woke up yesterday to the sounds of a woman throwing up for fifteen straight minutes. It might've been the woman who lives next door. Vomiting seems to come with the territory in India. And vomiting is not one consistent sound. If someone says to you, "I just heard a note from a piano", you'd have to ask, "was it a C sharp? Was it from the high end of the piano or the deep end? Was it loud, soft, long, staccato? For fifteen minutes this woman played for me a complete symphony. The deepest recesses of her throat were the most beautiful instruments I had ever heard.

Which brings me to yoga. I'm not an athlete (but I was a mathlete in school). I'm not flexible, pliable, and my back muscles aren't ripped and shredded. I've never stood in my head. And I get embarassed when I hear people chant for religious reasons. So, practicing yoga in India becomes a story of humiliation, weakness, disappointment, and frustration for me. And I'm only on my second class here. Some of the things hard for me so far:

1. Worst in Class. In class, I'm the first one who was forced to stop. There's about 100 people at my level (beginner). The moves start off fairly easy, and then get harder and harder. Saraswathi, the daughter of Pattabhi Jois, is leading the class. About 45 minutes in she looks over at me. I'm drenched in sweat. Everything hurts. The other people in the class are shining like gods, their sweat illuminating the etches of their brilliant muscles. I smell like gutter. Saraswathi looks over at me, "you stop now." So I'm the first to stop.

2. Everyone Looks at Me. I have to stay until the end of the class because we all do the closing moves together. So I'm sitting there not sure what to do. I'm in the back of the class. There's one move where everyone twists around. When I say "twist around" its almost like a science fiction movie where the aliens twist around their waist 360 degrees in order to make sure there's no danger. So everyone is twisting around in this impossible position, looking straight at me, the one guy in the back of the room not doing the move. Is this fair? Do I look back at them? Should I pretend I'm the teacher and they are all looking back at me for approval? Instead, I look down and act like I'm meditating.

3. The Men in The Class Are Perfect. I'm the only guy in the class who keeps my shirt on. Which is why I mention above I smell like gutter. Its worse than that though. I smell like something is dead in the walls of your house. The other guys take their shirts off. They have tattoos of dragons on their backs and crawling up their arms. They have muscles in places called tibias, femurs, psoas. Parts of the body I never heard of. Like when you suddenly look at a map of the world and realize for the first time that Africa is broken up into many tiny countries that you never knew existed and most likely will never visit.

4. My Secret Revealed. There was a move where both teaching assistants and Saraswathi had to come over and put me in position. I knew that they knew my secret then. That I was just pretending to be here. One woman pushing my back down. The other woman whispering urgently, relax your arm and stretch it out this way. Saraswathi saying, "leg wants go here!" My leg had never taken directions before. It never wanted anything before. I was praying at the time, "just let the fingers from my left hand clasp the fingers from my right hand behind me so they could leave."

5. Yoga Vision. Today I was waiting outside for Claudia to finish her class. Today was my "rest day". The advanced class was waiting to go in so there were about 40 advanced level students and me waiting outside. They all looked at me when I showed up. I was the special guest. Yoga supposedly makes your eyes shine brighter. This is what Claudia tells me. All of the advanced students looked at me with their x-ray vision. Their heat vision. I melted into the dust.

6. Sanskrit. At breakfast at a local restaurant there were no Indians. Only yoga students, still glistening from the sweat of their practice. Everyone was comparing notes on their class. "I had trouble with the full stretch on Utthita Hasta Padangusthasana". "I finally got past Ardha Baddha Padma Paschimottanasana". It seemed like everyone was fluent in some sort of yoga-ized Sanskrit. They all ordered things like granola. I had two orders of pancakes with bananas inside. Mmmm. It was good.

7. Chanting. At the beginning of class there's a chant. It starts off with a big "Ommmm". I can handle that. But then it goes into something else that I can't understand. Everyone else is doing the chant. For some reason I blush and I try to hum along with it but then blush more because why am I even humming?

8. Earnestness. People say things like, "its good its crowded here. More people in the world are doing yoga." They are earnest about it and everyone is agreeing. I'm not sure how to respond. Maybe, "I feel like world peace might be right around the corner." Or, "If only everyone had a fully developed tibia muscle less people might get divorced."

9. Coconuts. After practice on the first day I was sweating so much I thought I would have no more water left in my body. "Drink coconut juice," Claudia said to me and there was a guy cutting coconuts right outside the class. "It will give you electrolytes." All of the other students were outside drinking coconut juice already. They knew the drill. We're monkeys from a million generations ago and we need our coconuts so we can mate and have children. But I don't like coconut juice so we leave the other students there, all filling up with electrolytes so they can laugh and flirt once again.

10. Cold Shower. After the first class I went home to take a shower. But I'm not quite used to the smell of the water here yet. I am saying this very politely. And I couldn't figure out how to get hot water. So I took a freezing cold shower and couldn't get the soap off my skin. So for the rest of the day I was scratching all over like a wild animal, leaving scratch marks everywhere, when the soap dried into my skin and mixed with the general grime and dust outside.

Its day four and I'm loving every minute of my trip here. Tomorrow is my third class

Second Act

After we returned from that Mysore trip we were lucky to have Sharath tour New York City, we attended one week of his led classes, this is what James had to say about it:

Completely Humiliated...Again:

I keep doing it to myself. In January I went to India with Claudia to do yoga for a few weeks. I was utterly humiliated in positions I never thought possible while hundreds of people looked on.

Well, it happened again. Since we got back from India I've been trying to do yoga three or four times a week. Claudia says that its really two or three, best case, but what does she know? Does she have an abacus there whenever I do a sun salutation?

So we signed up for a one week class with Sharath Jois, whose grandfather, Pattabhi Jois, started Ashtanga Yoga and now Sharath is "the guy" since his grandfather passed away. Sharath was going to be in NYC for one week.

The first day we got there early. I was feeling a little better than in January because now I was more experienced. Three months more experienced. But I knew I was in trouble when the girl next to me was doing headstands just to "prepare" for the session.

At first, no problem. Sharath was walking around the room of 200 and giving the orders of what positions to be in and then counting the breaths. Five breaths on each position. I secretly hoped at the end of the class he'd walk up to Claudia and me and say, "hey, we should all grab dinner and become great friends."

Finally, out of the two hundred people, one of them needed help getting into a position. Me. On each breath in a stretch, Sharath had to push me lower, until my back was going to break in half. For some reason, I felt an abnormal urge to cry. Me. A grown man. Claudia says Sharath knows exactly how far he can push someone.

Then we finally reached a point where I couldn't do the positions anymore. Claudia was sitting next to me. She had both legs behind her neck and was leaning all the way to the floor so her nose was touching the floor. What the hell is that? Claudia had told me earlier I could "modify" the difficult positions until I was comfortable. How do I modify that? I just started sitting there figuring there must be other people like me. Behind us was a 90 year old woman. Her legs were behind her neck and her nose was touching the floor. As were the other 200 people in the room except for me. I felt depressed and a little ashamed.

Still, I tried to keep up. In my entire life I had never sweat so much. And the positions kept getting more and more brutal but I was able to do the moves that transition you into each position. At one point I saw that the regular yoga instructor that Claudia and I usually go to was about two mats over from me. Even he was just a student here. So what the hell was I doing here?

My glasses were so covered in sweat I couldn't see anything. Every other guy had their shirt off and, as usual, they had tattoos etched across every muscle. There was zero chance I was talking my shirt off not matter how wet with sweat it got. At one point you had to bring your legs straight up and your head and back straight up so your nose met your knees. Sharath had to help me grab my legs because they kept falling back to the ground. I can't even imagine what my face looked like. Red, sweaty, strained, crying, my legs flailing, my arms desperately trying to catch my toes before they fell again. 43 year olds can have heart attacks you know!

Afterwards, Claudia asked me how it went. I could barely walk. My arms were shaking. I was still sweating, and I couldn't stop my eyes from tearing like I was a little baby.

Today I'm going back for the second class.

In Conclusion

I offer here his accounts because they seemed to reassure a lot of people that a) he keeps it real b) it may be hard but it can be fun, and c) Myself -and every reader I know of- identifies with him, no matter what level, and we can all laugh together.

TWELVE: IF YOU WOULD LIKE TO TEACH ASHTANGA YOGA

My Own Authorization Story: You Can't Always Get What You Want

I wanted to be Authorized and Certified. That was my new year resolution in 2006. To be granted permission to teach Ashtanga yoga. By India. The real people. The place where the Guru lived. The place where permission was granted.

At that time authorization to teach this system was somewhat predictable. You had to go Mysore in South India four times (4 years in a row) for at least three months each time, and if lucky, you could receive authorization. The blessing.

Then you had to go four more times for 3 to 6 months to be certified. You were never supposed to ask for it or

Claudia Azula Altucher

even expect to get it. It was all a big mysterious and fascinating ordeal that meant your life was about to change. Big time.

I liked houses back then and I had just gotten myself one. I'll tell you about my house. It was a two-bedroom in a tree-lined street where only one or two cars would drive by every day.

I thought a house was a good investment, and the real estate agent put 1000 dollars of her own money to help with the down-payment. But of course I did not know that having a house involved raking the leaves in the Fall and shoveling snow in the Winter.

I did not like raking or shoveling because the yard and the drive-way were big. Too big.

Another "big" were my plans. I had an Excel chart with specific details of when I would go to India and for how long and it plotted events all the way to 2016.

I did not know where the money would come because I had just heard a big spiritual teacher say that "the money would come from wherever it was at the moment". So I did not worry about the money. Instead I plotted away in the little excel boxes, planning dates and numbers away, charting what was to happen.

Today I noticed that some things did not go exactly as planned.

In the Spreadsheet I was to be authorized last July. As in last summer, as in 2010. That is a long time ago and it did not happen at all. Furthermore when I scrolled to what was supposed to be happening today I found myself back in India and in my fourth trip, which I also had to cross down because I just returned from my second trip and would not even embark on the third one until 2012.

The biggest oversight in the chart is kapotasana, a very difficult pose of the intermediate series that one only gets to when the back is very flexible and after one is able to drop back from a standing position all the way to the floor into a bridge position. In "paper" I got kapotasana in March of 2010. That had me laughing because I spent all of 2010 -as in the whole year- trying to drop back. Which brings me back to kapotasana. What was I thinking?

Other things that were not on the chart did happen between then and now:

All doors of heaven opened up and made way so I could take 5 weeks off from my job. Twice! In America that is the bigger than a miracle. It is the impossible made possible.

On the first long absence I went to Mysore -early 2008 and much later than planned-, and in spite of my boss not being too happy about it.

The second extended absence took me to Thailand for more focused and dedicated practice time. I also got married and my father died. I lost a sister to life and gained two step-daughters who enjoy practicing yoga and making art projects with me, at least sometimes. I lost the job where I created the spreadsheet -on the exact day I returned from Thailand- and yes, the house with the big yard is also gone, thank you very much.

During my 2nd trip to Mysore I heard again and again that I must do my yoga, and that all would come. I hated hearing that because I always knew what I wanted and I really did not need a person of yet another country to tell me what I wanted. I lived in lots of Countries. And besides, I had a chart.

But one night, not so long ago and when I was back in the comfort of my own bed, in my beautiful rented house that needs no raking, I wondered: What if yoga was supposed to just put me in touch with what my own spirit wants to express, and once that happened then all doors would open, and then all would indeed come?

If I could talk back to the woman I was in 2006, all excited and happy over the Excel spreadsheet, I would tell her to keep those exact same goal, because it was that chart that brought me to where I am today. Different, yet great. Surrendering feels good.

"It takes time and patience; everyone wants to be a teacher without even being a student. The shala gets calls from people asking how they can become teachers; the answer: Do your practice"
Sharath Jois in Conference, March of 2011

About Authorization and Certification

It is advised to travel to Mysore for the experience of it and to further surrender to the practice. Not seeking authorization or certification. Once we have our own agenda it stops being yoga. That should not stop anyone from making Excel spreadsheets though. They are fun and have their place, but remember, once we leave the planning mode we work at being present and with what is.

You can read all about the institute's regulations in their website www.kpjayi.org.

THIRTEEN: PERMISSION GRANTED

Many people coming into Ashtanga Yoga wonder about their own abilities because of their age, health, state of mind, state of affairs in their lives. Permission is one of those things we all struggle with.

To this, I would first remind everyone of what Pattabhi Jois would say repeatedly: *Anyone can practice, old, sick, very old, there is only one person that cannot, that is the lazy!*

Granting Ourselves Permission

In October of 2007 I told my boss that I needed five weeks off to go to India. His heart skipped a bit. He said that in America asking for even two weeks is a lot. Three months later and five minutes before boarding Emirates flight 204 to Dubai/Bangalore, that same boss text-ed me a last minute message on the company blackberry: Have fun!

I gave myself permission to go to India. It was a directive from Spirit. The outer world had no choice but to comply because I was coming from a position of center and power, it was just what needed to happen and so it did.

Isn't permission one of those things that leave us wondering about our abilities in the world? Don't we all lose sleep over having the "right qualifications" "authorizations" "certifications" "blessings" "acknowledgments" "degrees"?

Therefore,

By appointment of the Royal Self, through the gateways of cosmic blessings, **you are now and forever given permission to**:

1. **Start Yoga**. Yes you can. Get to the front of the mat, do what you can, find a class that you like, go ahead.

2. **Plug Leaks in Your Life**. Find the areas where energy is leaking. Ashtangis would call this: "Tighten your anus" or "use mulabandha". Think of it in terms of:

    *   Who is that person that is draining your energy in every phone-call? Get rid of him/her if possible and at all costs.

    *   Where is your time going? How much Facebook? How Much TV?

- Where is your money going? Create a beautiful and realistic budget.

- Is your room/home in order? make it so.

- Are you gossiping? if so, consider not doing so for a while and seeing how it feels. Gossip is one of the biggest leaks, and that is a well-kept secret. Now you know.

1. **Treat Yourself To Real Rest**. You deserve it. Yes even if you lost your job and have one billion responsibilities. "No sleep no prana". I said that. Because I can. And because I know is true.

2. **Set Aside "ME" Time**, no dogs, no cats, no turtles, no kids, no husband/wife, just You. See if you like the company you keep, or if there are some areas of you that you need to make friends with.

3. **Believe**. You have way much more to give the world than you think you do. Now that the plugs are in place and the energy is being kept within you, re-direct it to creativity. Speak to your soul, ask what it wants from you.

4. **Know That You Are Loved**, wanted, and on purpose. Because you are. You are here right now because your own unique way of expressing and synthesizing life is a gift to the world. It can only come from you. Let's start by giving it some respect.

5. **You Know That Dream?** that old dream you have of starring in a play? writing that novel? traveling around the world? Fill in the blank? That one that keeps popping up and invites you to try. You are now allowed to do it. Start it.

Take the first step in faith. You don't have to see the whole staircase, just take the first step.
Martin Luther King.

6. **Vanish Naysayers.** Once and for all. They did not read this book yet, so it is understandable they will not like it when you begin connecting with spirit and changing. Bless them, and keep going. More importantly, don't try to change them, it will be of no use, let them go through their own path, be they ready when they might. Just focus on your path.

7. **Start a Blog.** Talk about your passions and find community. Blogs have the power of getting us interconnected and talking about the things we love to talk about, uncensored, in the raw. Just remember the only rule of blogging: be true to yourself and never be mean to others.

8. **Trust Yourself.** Unequivocally, wholeheartedly, fiercely. Whatever happens today, in whichever way you respond, say to yourself that you did the best thing with the knowledge you have at this moment. It is all working out. Trust it. It is.

9. **Speak Up.** Nobody can read your mind, at least not for now, in this time of ultra information, so say what it is that you like and what it is that bothers you. Express it to make your life a better representation of your own integrity. No need to nag or be annoying but all the need in the world to keep it real.

10. **Love Your So-Called Imperfections.** Whatever it is you are not happy with about your body about send it love. Remember that it is what makes you unique. Get in the habit of saying 'Oh you are hot'! every time you catch your image in a mirror or passing window.

11. **Put the House in Order**, one room per weekend if the whole place sounds too daunting. While at it, give things away you do not use anymore. Create space for new beginnings. New Spaces, more air, more room. You deserve it.

12. **Cook Something Nutritious** and wonderful for yourself, include dessert. You are allowed to nurture yourself, you are allowed to eat. Trust your body.

13. **Play.** Is not that hard. Go visit people with kids if you do not have any. They know how to do it. Take notes, because you are now allowed and granted full permission to play. So make sure to

remember. Also, consider that adults are just bigger kids. I know I am.

14. **Ask God** out loud and clear to guide you in this new emergent God/Goddess coming through you. Tell God that your creativity will be expressed, you will put in the work, but what comes out is his or her work, you are just the channel. Then let it flow through you. Try it.

15. **Remember That We Want to be Happy,** not authorized, certified, PhD-ed, rich, famous, or otherwise recognized by some outside authority. You want to connect with your own truth and let it shine.

16. **Dare** to do something new today. Put on that purple wig, paint your toe-nails blue (I just did). Say "thank you but I will pass" if you don't want to go to that event. Take the evening off to yourself to just read that book you love.

17. **Create an Encouraging Banner** and hang it on your wall where you will see it every day. Mine reads "Yes I can" and is hanged on the room of the house where I practice yoga-asanas. Why? It reassures me. I have seen people create a banner that says: "Believe", or "Endless Possibilities", or "I am flowing with creative ideas". What is yours?

18. **Write 3 things You Grant Others Permission to Do**. Giving others permission has an effect akin to

that of being happy for others when something good happens to them. It opens us, it sends our minds the signal that there is plenty. It can also be pretty revealing when it comes to the things we would like to give permission to our own selves.

19. **Gratitude.** List all the people and things you are grateful for in your life. Do not forget your eyes, legs, hands, ability to read, children, family. Look at that list. It will probably be very, very long. Say thank you. Often.

20. **Notice** where you are. You are standing in a little, tiny planet, that is spinning very fast, in the middle of a vast universe. What you see is not all really real but a constant orchestration of universal forces, a symphony of natural forces. You do not ever have to believe everything your mind says. Things are ephemeral and changing all the time, the only thing that is real is that connection you feel right now with the creator, with your spirit, let it be, let it through.

Whether you think "you can" or "you can't" either way you are
right.
Henry Ford.

FOURTEEN: 9 LAME EXCUSES THAT KEEP PEOPLE AWAY FROM YOGA

Have you ever heard someone tell you that they would like to start a yoga practice but: "fill in the blank"? Excuses seem to abound.

A friend of mine recently asked me about the common excuses I have heard and even though at first I didn't want to think about it, I confess that eventually I found a certain almost evil pleasure in coming up with the list, had so much fun I even made a video with extra excuses that are not even in it:

What is your excuse?

1.-Don't Know The Poses

When my uncle (who is now 60) was about to attend his first day of elementary school he hid under the bed and cried because: "he did not know how to write or read". I found that cute, provided that we are six years old, of course.

2.-Don't Want To Take My Shirt Off

Most of the men in class keep a short and a t-shirt on, some get over heated and take the top off, but there is no code of conduct that determines whether one has to wear one.

3.-I'm Not Flexible

Pattabhi Jois said it all when he utter these words: "Body is not stiff, mind is stiff". You can hear it in your head with an Indian accent, it sounds more profound.

When you make the shift and notice that flexibility is in the mind then a whole new world opens, you can be more present for any pose you may be doing and just by opening the mind you can immediately notice the better breathing, better disposition and deeper reach. You may have an *aha!* Moment and realize you are more flexible than you *thought*.

4.-I Don't Want To Chant

Fair enough, many classes start with one simple Aum at the beginning. Ashtanga yoga has a whole chant, but not all styles adhere to this. Also noticing our feelings around things that make us uncomfortable is a great meditation. For example: can we remain equanimous?

Who would have thought that through this we can get started with our work on the other branches of yoga? We can start observing what the mind tells us around chanting, we can just notice our reactions.

5.-I Want a Real Workout

I can understand this. Some yoga classes are very slow, but not all of them are like that, there is a class for every level of intensity, flexibility and courage (if I dare say so). Just playing the DVD of Mark Darby for example, the one with the primary series, is work, a lot of work. Try it if you do not believe me, just the standing sequence is enough to get the blood, muscles, and the breath going.

6.-I'm Not Fit Enough

Yeah, nothing to worry about, we are all very self-conscious and nobody thinks they are fit enough anyway, so coming along is a show of camaraderie.

7.-Have No Money

Yoga can be practiced at home with a DVD that costs no more than 20 dollars or so. Classes, of course, are a great way to get corrections and inspiration and, if possible, always recommended.

8.-Have No Time

There are short classes, especially in gyms. You can also leave classes earlier, although teachers tend not to like that, but you can make an arrangement. People in the yoga world understand, they are approachable. If you do happen to leave a class early always remember to do savasana (corpse/relaxation pose) before re-entering normal paced life, your nervous system will thank you with extra years of life.

9- It Will Take Years To Do Those Impressive Asanas

Maybe, maybe not. There are a few really cool looking asanas that can be mastered rather quickly, for example: The whole Sun Salutation sequence or even the shoulder-stands. I know it "looks" difficult, but it is not, and pretty much every class includes an attempt, so you will build up fast and impress the yogi out of all your friends.

By the way, I made an animated video over the excuses that keep people from doing yoga, see it here:

http://www.youtube.com/watch?v=rJFik0ozfQs&feature=player_embedded

FIFTEEN: THINGS I HAVE LEARNED RECENTLY FROM SHARATH JOIS

I find that Sharath is transitioning into *Guru* status in his own right through dedication, his commitment to practice and teaching, his utter determination to pass along what he learned and his invitation to all of us to put the practice into action where it counts.

These are some of the things he has said at recent conferences I attended either in Mysore or in NYC which inspired me and helped me along the path. This chapter includes notes taken by me and with my own view of things, at times I paraphrase because perhaps I did not take down word by word what he was saying.

His main message, no matter when or where is always an invitation to find the guru within, **"do your practice, the right answer will come to you"**, **"do your practice, all is coming"**, **"do yoga"**. He has what we in the west call a "media message", and this is it. He repeats it every time and every where.

This is the brightest indication of how important it is for us to hear it, again and again, process it, understand it and connect with our spiritual source daily, trusting that the rest does take care of itself, because it does.

"Once you are true you do not need to fear"

And so it is, once we know what our source spirit directive is then, as Gurji would say: "why fear?".

We do our practice, that is what allows us to be true, to establish the connection, to come clean to ourselves, to eliminate the drama, to trust that we are on the right path, to believe that we are on it for a reason, to surrender, to thrive.

"Practice should be with respect faith and over a long period of time."

Sharath often discusses the importance of sticking to the technique explained in the scriptures, in the proper way, to respect the tradition and the teachings of the lineage. He uses the example of "pujas" or Indian ways of praying to God and how they have a specific format and practice and that our practice, says Sharath, is just like it, it has its system.

Pattabhi Jois was an example of dedication. He used to drive every day to the old yoga shala at 4:15 in the morning and again in the afternoons. He taught for long periods of time often not even eating anything until late in the afternoon.

When talking about **faith** he told us at a recent conference that yes, it is important to have faith. It does not matter what God you believe in because God is one, but faith is necessary.

When someone questioned him about **doubt** in our practice he said that we need to get "grounded in the practice, do it for the love of it, not for the next pose, not for the authorization, but because it works".

We do it for a long period of time, and when we have doubts that is usually when we get the best practice - should we choose to stick with it-. *"Everyone has doubts at some point,"* Sharath said. *"I had doubts."*

On the subject of **greed** he said that instead of focusing on the next pose, focus on perfecting what you have. Perfection of the primary series is very important.

When discussing **injury** he said *"You have to be intelligent"* and don't force things, you know what to do, how far you can go. And asana slows with age, but we always do asana.

He even gave the example of when Pattabhi Jois got very sick in the 90s and how as soon as he was out of the hospital he would walk to the hallway of his home holding on to the walls (could not be touched for assistance when doing his puja) and go do his prayers, his Gayatri mantra, his other chants. Always doing his practice.

And on the subject of **rest**, he pointed that Asana should go on for no more than 2 hours, otherwise: "*You can go crazy*". The only 3 yoga sutras dealing with asana are set on calming the mind, not over-exciting it.

During my second trip to Mysore I made it a point of taking notes during each conference and afterwards writing about it because I thought it worth-wile to share the message with other practitioners.   Even after I left I had other practitioners send me their notes on conferences where I could not be present. All those posts can be found here:

http://earthyogi.blogspot.com/search/label/Conference

SIXTEEN: 18 SUGGESTIONS TO IMPROVE YOUR YOGA PRACTICE

I came up with these suggestions based on a series developed at the blog, it is mostly tips that I use here and there, not meant to be taken all at once, but that if taken, say, one at the time, or choosing one a day, can result in a deeper experience of the asana practice and the whole of yoga.

1. Learning the opening and closing chants. See resources.

2. Slowing down, taking five counts for the in-breath and five for the out breath. I tried this for a couple of weeks during my Mysore morning practice and found that it brought me a lot more in touch with the body I ever imagined it would

3. Taking a led class.

4. Reading the Yoga Sutras. See resources.

5. Checking on nutrition. Are you getting enough nutrients? greens? salads? juices?. Nutrition is a very important part of the practice and your success in it as well as in life will be determined by the quality and quantity of the food you eat.

Food must be eaten in measured quantities. It must be very pure.
T. Krishnamacharya. Yoga Makaranda

6. Savasana (Corpse pose). Are you giving your body enough time to rest and cool down after practice?

Here is what Krishnamacharya says about rest:

"After completing their yoga practice consisting of asana and pranayama, the yoga practitioner must rest for fifteen minutes keeping the body on the floor before coming outside. If you come outdoors soon after completing yogabhyasa [practice], the breeze will enter the body through the minute pores on the skin and cause many kinds of disease. Therefore, one should stay inside until the sweat subsides, rub the body nicely and sit contentedly and rest for a short period"

7. Saturday practice, or a Castor oil bath. See chapter on it.

8. Learning the names of all the poses of the primary series.

9. Focusing on inversions. Learning about them, their benefits, their power.

10. Attending a workshop.

11. Internal cleansing. Here are five easy methods:

    http://earthyogi.blogspot.com/2010/10/5-simple-yogic-cleansings.html

12. Food fast. When I visited Mysore the thing that called my attention the most about advanced practitioners is how little they ate, and how some attended indian treatments from the ayurvedic school that recommended fasting. Of course this is not to be taken lightly and must be done with full awareness and under close and experienced supervision. It is a suggestion here, as in something to investigate further.

13. Media fast. The title says it all, no news, for a week. Refreshing.

14. Mantras. Learning and chanting them is very powerful, but I can only speak from my own experience. The Gayatri Mantra for example, has enormous benefits and Guruji used to sing it 108 times a day, every day. – See resources.

15. Making a list of things that we are grateful for and keeping it where we can see it, remembering it often.

16. Offering our practice for the benefit of all beings

17. Getting a massage. I am very fond of massages, especially the deep tissue ones.

18. Surrendering. To the practice, to doing it every day, to the commitment it takes, to gratitude for having found it.

SEVENTEEN: UNUSUAL YOGA QUOTES THAT JOLT ME BACK INTO CENTER

I like quotes and noticed that lots of them have been overused, so I went on a search for the ones that really do it for me, the ones that give me energy and came up with these. Most of them come from recognized yogis, others from authors that you may not think of as yogis, but that probably were or are.

1. Married life is 7th Series. -*Pattabhi Jois*

2. No coffee no prana. -*Sharath Jois*

3. Turn on the lights of the pose. -*Richard Freeman*

4. Why hurry? –*Sharath Jois*

5. Let your speech be true and sweet. – *Krishnamacharya*

6. Before you've practiced, the theory is useless. After you've practiced, the theory is obvious. - *David Williams*

7. Never be in debt. Never reside near enemies. Never trap your body through disease. Never forget the Lord with his consort who resides in the heart. -*Krishnamacharya*

8. Don't just do something, sit there! -*Unknown*

9. If your compassion does not include yourself, it is incomplete.- *Jack Kornfield*

10. Our deepest fear is not that we are inadequate. Our deepest fear is that we are powerful beyond measure. It is our light, not our darkness that most frightens us. We ask ourselves, Who am I to be brilliant, gorgeous, talented, fabulous? Actually, who are you not to be?.- *Marianne Williamson*

11. Don't drawn in a glass of water. *Spanish saying*

12. When one experiences truth, the madness of finding fault with others disappears. -*S.N.Goenka*

13. All that we are is the result of what we have thought. *Buddha*

14. A fool thinks himself to be wise, but a wise man knows himself to be a fool. -*William Shakespeare*

15. The first wealth is health. *-Ralph Waldo Emerson*

16. To one established in non-stealing all wealth comes. *-Patanjali*

17. Health, longevity, a tranquil mind. –T. *Krishnamacharya (from A.G. Mohan's book "Krishnamacharya, His Life and Teachings" when asked the question: What is important in life?).*

18. I refer to the Yoga Makaranda -the Tamil translation- Whenever I want to just shut up and listen to my Guru Krishnamacharya – *S. Ramaswami*

19. There's a saying that poets and women should never be coerced... Similarly never use force in teaching or practicing asana - *T. Krishnamacharya*

EIGHTEEN: A FEW WAYS TO PRACTICE YOGA WHEN WE ARE OFF THE MAT

If you do asana but then go and punch someone in the face,
then what is the point of practice?
Sharath Jois

Most of our yoga happens when we step off the mat because that is when the real challenges of life occur. The beginning of the exploration of the other limbs of yoga happens as we interact with others, and in how we treat them and ourselves.

Consider these suggestions as you go through your day

Not stealing, following the Yoga Sutras when they say that by abstaining from taking what does not belong to us, and that also means not stealing other's time, or energies.

Cooking/eating right, meaning lots of greens, lean proteins, you know the drill

Exercising contentment, living like a yogi in the midst of worldly matters. Practicing being in a state of equanimity and stopping the preconditioned reactions we tend to have all the time.

Loving ourselves, in every possible way.

Conserving our sexual energy, See the chapter on yogis ways of finding the man or woman of your dreams

Being truthfull, always

Not killing

Praying

Practicing concentration

Thinking "**how can I help**"

Thinking "**how can I add value**"

Feeling our emotions, neurosis and fears, and not reacting because of them in any way that hurts others

Taking responsibilities for our lives and never playing victim again

Keeping our word. When we say we will do something, that needs to be respected like a law, it must happen, otherwise we are dishonoring our inborn power of manifestation. It might be small, but just like Warren Buffet does not bet a mere dollar in a silly game, neither should we use our words on promises we do not intend to keep

Speaking with a clean vocabulary, never using bad words

Being kind, always

Respecting teachers

Respecting everyone

Giving credit where it is due

Being grateful, often, and for everything, including the ability to discern, to read, to see, to walk, to smell, to move

Giving, even if in prayer form, making it a habit to give something to everyone we encounter. It can be as big as doing all their laundry or as small as a prayer: "may you be happy"

De cluttering, making space, sacred space

Respecting our own psychological constitution and working with it, always starting where we are, with the intention to move towards center

NINETEEN: WHY DO BILLIONAIRES PRACTICE ASHTANGA YOGA?

You could argue that people that have spent their whole life accumulating billions are not precisely just type A personalities, but rather type AAA+, or more. Once they did achieve such level of wealth what do they have left to worry about? Yes, you guessed right: losing it. There are two ways they can lose all that wealth, either:

> a) the world ends, or
>
> b) they die

Some billionaires are very focused on saving the world, which is a great thing, they are somewhat protectors like Bill Gates or Warren Buffet who have donated more money than any government or individual before them and in the history of the world to help.

Then there are other types of billionaires who are also doing good for the world but they are just as much focused on living a long and healthy life. These individuals have all the money and mind/research power at their disposal to find out the best way to stay healthy, and some of them happen to have chosen Ashtanga yoga. They are:

Paul Tudor Jones. Estimated net worth 3.2 B. Founder of Tudor Investment Corporation from Greenwhich CT.   He is also the husband of Sonia Jones, who has now teamed up with the Jois family and created Jois Yoga [JoisYoga.com] centers in Greenwich, CT, Encinitas, CA, and Sydney, Australia.

Daniel Loeb. Estimated worth 3.6 B. Not only is he a dedicated practitioner that raises every day at 5:30 to get on the mat, he also travels to Mysore from time to time.

William H. Gross. Estimated net worth 1.3B. He reportedly practices ashtanga 5 times a week and has said that "his best ideas come when he is standing on his head".

I actually do not need the research anymore as I can tell by the effects of the practice in my life that I am in the right path, but I thought I would share this curious detail with you because it certainly caught my imagination when I first heard about it.

TWENTY: WHAT IS NEXT?

What is next is integrating the other limbs of yoga.

By now you are probably under the clear understanding that asana is the beginning of the thread but eventually, and with practice, curiosity for the other branches will be awakened.

If you find yourself here this is the moment to start reading the Yoga Sutras of Patanjali –see resources-.

If you want to put it in practice try and discriminate every thought you get and strive to stay away from sending all your energy into them, rather focus on just being, with no mental commentary.

When the hunger for more strikes perhaps a good starting point is also to further explore the yamas and niyamas and pay especial attention to how your actions affect you and others around you.

Further along, the fourth limb of yoga is pranayama – breath extension-. Pattabhi Jois was known for teaching it to his students back in the day, but as the years went by he made an executive decision to stop that practice and in his last days he was known for saying that nobody should take pranayama until solidly established in asana. By solidly established he meant third series. This could be just a legend, I never actually heard him say that in person, but it is the word on the street. The best thing to do might be to talk to your teacher about it.

I have been practicing pranayama in other traditions I there are many teachers around the world that offer training in it and do it well. I invite you to visit the book club at the blog to read more about it.

Pratyahara is the next limb. Normally explained as "withdrawing the senses", Sharath recently talked about it beautifully in one of his latest conferences in Encinitas. He said: *"When everything you see is seen as divine, everything you hear, heard as divine, everything touched felt as divine, then you have reached pratyahara"*.

After *Pratyahara* is possible, then *concentration* follows, which, I hear –as I have not yet experienced it- leads to *meditation* and eventually to *Samadhi*. Thoughts on the other limbs of yoga are always interesting but beyond the scope of this book.

When all else fails, just feel the life in you and become present with what is, that is the final destination.

TWENTY-ONE: 32 UNUSUAL WAYS TO LOVE OURSELVES

I happen to think that loving ourselves is the very first principle for anything in life. Without self-love it is difficult to love others, or to give, or to embark on any new adventure.

Although it sounds selfish and counterintuitive self-love is the only way in which we can learn how to love another one. Seeing what is good in us is the fundamental principle behind seeing what is good in everyone, in recognizing our own divinity and hence others' divinities.

Warning, this might lead to better self-esteem at worst and the realization that we are all divine beings at best.

1. Learning to say "*thank you but I think I will skip*" when we do not want to do something

2. Taking responsibility for how we feel

3. Using only positive and glorious words when talking about ourselves

4. Before eating asking "*what is the healthiest most nutritious thing I can eat now*"?, then trusting

what we hear, really trusting. May be ice-cream today, might be spinach tomorrow, if we trust.

5. Taking a media fast once in a while

6. Taking a "me" day off, for real

7. Praying at home, in the train, in the car, during laundry, after yoga, on the street, in the shower, etc.

8. Taking a long walk, with only ourselves

9. Remembering our priorities

10. Honoring those whom we love, and our teachers

11. Using place mats and the art of conversation during meals

12. *The kitchen sink is always empty and clean.* This has become a mantra for me.

13. Making the bed every morning

14. Taking a Saturday afternoon for a beauty treatment

15. Writting down ten things we would like to experience in this lifetime

16. Looking at the list often

17. Reaching out to someone we know needs it

18. Giving something away

19. Speaking half the times we think we need to

20. Organizing the closet

21. Buying clothes only if they fit 2 criteria: 1) comfortable, and 2) makes me feel fabulous

22. Avoiding drama at all costs

23. But 22 does not mean we avoid dealing with issues we know we need to deal with

24. Speaking up when is necessary

25. Learning to be compassionate towards others but also, and most importantly, to ourselves

26. Going to bed at around the same time every night

27. Making sure we go to the bathroom for number 1 and number 2 every day

28. Looking at our reflection and going "Wow you are hot!"

29. Appreciating that it really does not need to be perfect, it just needs to be

30. Using our energy efficiently

31. Sending love towards the Earth

32. Playing. Often

RESOURCES

Learning the Opening and Closing Chants

- Here is **Pattabhi Jois singing the opening chant**: http://kpjayi.org/the-practice/opening-prayer you can also read it and see what it means. And here is the **closing prayer**: http://kpjayi.org/the-practice/closing-prayer

- **Manju Jois has a CD** that includes the opening and closing mantras.

    http://www.ashtanga.com/html/p.lasso?p=10137

- Also, visit **www.kpjayi.org** for the history of Ashtanga, pictures, bios, etc.

Suggested DVDs To Start Practicing

Of course nothing replaces getting to a studio and learning directly from a more advanced practitioner than us. Forming a relationship with a good teacher is the recommended way to go, always.

To find a teacher near you visit the AYRI website and click on teachers [http://kpjayi.org/teachers-directory/asia]. Make sure to also research the studios in your area to see if there are any Mysore programs as sometimes teachers do not go on the list in the website right away.

There are also many teachers who are not yet authorized/certified but that are very good and can help you. It is all about how you feel when you are in the class.

It is important that you can feel safe and confident that you are being led and supported. And remember, the best test to see if yoga is working for you is that your life will get better. Just do not rush things and give it a few years. Yes, years.

Teachers tend to tour quite a bit so keep an eye on the internet for upcoming workshops that may be coming to your town. Ashtanga.com keeps a very updated list.

If you do not have access to a teacher there are some alternatives in DVD. I have not watched all of them nor do I know the full story behind them, I am just relating to you my own experience and pointing to resources that have helped me or other practitioners I have spoken with.

Richard Freeman

Is a senior teacher with many over 40 years of experience and a direct student of Sri K. Pattabhi Jois. He has been a certified student for a long time. He has 2 critical DVDs that are excellent resources for learning the primary series. One is called *Yoga with Richard Freeman: An Introduction to Ashtanga Yoga* and the other one is *Yoga with Richard Freeman: Ashtanga Yoga The Primary Series*.

Richard uses many metaphors when teaching that have done wonders during my first attempts at the primary series. For example, during prasarita padottanasana he asks students to *"turn on the lights of the pose"*. You could actually think of that on any pose and it would help you remember to engage the whole body, the bandhas, get centered, breathe deeper. At least it did for me.

You can also visit his website's store where he has a wealth of other resources like studio talks, tapes on breathing etc.

http://yogaworkshop.com/store/store.php

Kino MacGregor

has two helpful introductory DVDs to start the practice of asanas to. One is called *Ashtanga Yoga Primary Series*, and a new one she just released is called: *Introduction to Ashtanga Yoga DVD with Kino*

MacGregor, Greg Nardi and Tim Feldmann . I have not seen this one yet as, at the time of this publication it has just been offered for sale, but the promo video says that it contains a brief explanation on breathing, one on the philosophy of Ashtanga yoga and then an abbreviated version of the primary series with adjustments. Here is the website's store.

http://kinoyoga.com/?product_type=dvd

Mark Darby

Ashtanga Yoga Primary Series DVD. If you speak French, this is the one to get, as you can have it play in English or *en Francais... oui.* There are two teachers in the video, Mark who is a certified student of Pattabhi Jois shows the full form while Nicole Bordeleau, his assistant teacher, demonstrates variations for people just coming into the practice.

Here is his website:
http://www.sattvayogashala.com/index.html

And the DVD: http://www.amazon.com/Ashtanga-Yoga-Primary-Mark-Darby/dp/B0006I036C?ie=UTF8&tag=earyog08-20&link_code=btl&camp=213689&creative=392969

Sharath Jois

has a few DVDs of the Primary Series. In my opinion they are great because he does not talk at all, rather he just sticks to the count, and,

should you ever visit Mysore this is what a led class would look like.

The one consideration is that the count is just as is, which could be a little fast from someone just coming into it. Other than that it is a great inspiration to practice with the teacher of teachers.

Sharath's website and store is here: http://kpjayi.org/resources/dvds

Manju Jois

Has a DVD called: Ashtanga Yoga Workshop.

http://www.ashtanga.com/html/p.lasso?p=10168

David Garrigues

has a DVD called: *The Ashtanga Primary series Led Instructed*. Just as the title suggest, he explains things as he counts and takes you through the primary series. See here:

http://www.amazon.com/David-Garrigues-Ashtanga-Primary-Instructed/dp/B004JHNAF2?ie=UTF8&tag=earyog08-20&link_code=btl&camp=213689&creative=392969

Basia Lipska

has an English/Polish DVD. I have not seen it but a reader of the blog tells me that it goes through the series with modifications.

http://www.ashtanga.com/html/p.lasso?p=10217

Lino Miele

is a very senior teacher that wrote a very impressive book on both the primary and intermediate series together with Pattabhi Jois –see books- He has a DVD on the primary series.
http://www.linomiele.com/media.html

Melanie Flower
http://www.ashtanga.com/html/p.lasso?p=10072

David Swenson

First Series DVD:

http://www.ashtanga.net/store/Practice-DVDs/CDs/c5/index.html?osCsid=r2nilc27k9nrcmhu9d1j06e8o4

John Scott

Ashtanga Yoga Primary Series:
http://www.amazon.com/Ashtanga-Yoga-Primary-John-Scott/dp/B000BFHDY0/ref=sr_1_2?ie=UTF8&qid=1304889999&sr=1-2-catcorr

On Anatomy

Yoga Anatomy DVD, Volumes 1 and 2, by David Keil

http://www.yoganatomy.com/dvd.html

Practice Cards

Some people love to have cheat sheets as they get started and as a way to remember what comes next. I know I did. Here is an extensive list to choose from:

http://www.ashtanga.com/html/action.lasso?-database=ygpricelist.fm&-layout=w&-response=sc_category.html&category=Posters%20and%20Practice%20Card&-search&-sortField=t1

Books to Read

Why so many? Different books speak to different people and personalities. It might be a good idea to get one or two and see how they feel. For my thoughts on them visit the blog: ClaudiaYoga.com

Yoga Mala by Sri K. Pattabhi Jois.

http://www.amazon.com/Yoga-Mala-Original-Teachings-Ashtanga/dp/0865477515/ref=sr_1_1?ie=UTF8&qid=1304890660&sr=8-1

Guruji A Portrait of Sri K. Pattabhi Jois Through the Eyes of His Students by Guy Donahaye and Eddie Stern. A great book with stories from students of the Guru from the early stages.

http://www.amazon.com/Guruji-Portrait-Pattabhi-Through-Students/dp/0865477493/ref=pd_sim_b_4

Ashtanga Yoga Practice and Philosophy, by Gregor Maehle.

http://www.amazon.com/Ashtanga-Yoga-Philosophy-Gregor-Maehle/dp/1577316061/ref=pd_sim_b_4

Ashtanga Yoga: The Practice Manual: An Illustrated Guide to Personal Practice, by David Swenson:

http://www.amazon.com/Ashtanga-Yoga-Practice-Illustrated-Personal/dp/1891252089/ref=pd_sim_b_3

Ashtanga Yoga: The Definitive Step-by-Step Guide to Dynamic Yoga by John Scott:

http://www.amazon.com/Ashtanga-Yoga-Definitive-Step-Step/dp/0609807862/ref=pd_sim_b_4

Ashtanga Yoga, by Lino Miele.

http://www.amazon.com/Ashtanga-Yoga-yoga-Lino-Miele/dp/5914780039/ref=sr_1_2?ie=UTF8&s=books&qid=1304890844&sr=1-2

The Mirror of Yoga: Awakening the Intelligence of Body and Mind, by Richard Freeman

http://www.amazon.com/dp/159030795X?tag=earyog08-20&camp=213761&creative=393545&linkCode=bpl&creativeASIN=159030795X&adid=12BB4AF3N10RAV5TTJQY&

Ashtanga Yoga As It Is, by Matthew Sweeney

Pranayama, The Breath Of Yoga, by Gregor Maehle.

http://www.amazon.com/Ashtanga-Yoga-As-Revised-Third/dp/0975780700/ref=sr_1_12?s=books&ie=UTF8&qid=1304890869&sr=1-12

Further Reading

It will happen, you will get curious as you go along, at least that is what happened to me. If you do, these are gems to start with:

The Bhagavad Gita

The Yoga Sutras of Patanjali

The Yoga Makaranda – by Sri Tirumalai Krishnamacharya. The best part is that you can download it for free:

https://docs.google.com/viewer?a=v&pid=explorer&chrome=true&srcid=0B7JXC_g3qGlWM2IyOWNlNWEtZmU1NC00NmM0LTg2OTEtNWQxMzg0NDVjMmU4&hl=en&authkey=CJDkxU4&pli=1

Krishnamacharya His Life and Teachings, by A.G. Mohan

http://www.amazon.com/Krishnamacharya-Life-Teachings-G-Mohan/dp/159030800X/ref=sr_1_1?s=books&ie=UTF8&qid=1304891430&sr=1-1

Magazines

Namarupa is a privately published magazine run by Eddie Stern -a senior teacher and certified student-, a very interesting read with great pictures.

http://www.namarupa.org/

Mantras

Learning the Gayatri Mantra. Sharath mentioned in one of his conferences that Pattabhi Jois used to recite this mantra 108 times per day. It is said to be the most auspicious mantra of all. You can read more about it at the blog.

To learn it see Srivatsa Ramaswami's page (Ramaswami was a student of Krishnamacharya for over 30 years).

http://vinyasakrama.com/Chants

Just For Fun

- **Sri K. Pattabhi Jois Ashtanga Yoga, Encinitas**, 3rd and 4th Series

  http://www.amazon.com/Pattabbi-Jois-Ashtanga-Encinitas-California/dp/B0007RK4GQ?ie=UTF8&tag=earyog08-20&link_code=btl&camp=213689&creative=392969

- David Swenson's **Ashtanga Yoga 2nd and 3rd Series**

  http://www.amazon.com/Ashtanga-Yoga-Practice-2nd-3rd/dp/B000GHK60G?ie=UTF8&tag=earyog08-20&link_code=btl&camp=213689&creative=392969

Documentary

- **Ashtanga Yoga New York** – A Yoga Documentary, directed by Mary Wigmore.

  http://www.amazon.com/Ashtanga-NY-Documentary-Willem-Dafoe/dp/B0002J4ZT6/ref=sr_1_1?s=dvd&ie=UTF8&qid=1304891870&sr=1-1

Your Resources:

Let me know if you have found other resources that helped you from a perspective of someone just coming into the practice.

KEEP IN TOUCH

I am always curious about yogis and enjoy the conversations that can be sparked, please comment at the blog www.ClaudiaYoga.com.

If you liked the book I would very much appreciate it if you could *like it on Amazon* and, should you feel inclined, *write a review* as well so that others can find it.

I am grateful for you reading.

If you would like to write to me, contact me in Twitter at Twitter.com/ClaudiaYoga

Let's talk.

ABOUT THE AUTHOR

Claudia Azula Altucher has studied yoga since 1999 in the traditions of Iyengar, Ashtanga, and Sivananda. Her research and practice focus since the year 2005 has been Ashtanga in the tradition of Sri K. Pattabhi Jois.

She has studied at the Ashtanga Yoga Research Institute in Mysore several times, and practices daily either at home or in NYC.

Claudia has also studied pranayama in Thailand at the Centered Yoga Institute and continues her research on this limb of yoga in the tradition of the Kaivalyahdama Institute of India. She has practiced meditation by sitting at Viapassana courses and these days tries to bring presence to everything, as a daily practice.

She believes that yoga expands beyond culture and language and has contributed to both Spanish and English blogs on yoga.

She writes daily at ClaudiaYoga.com. You can follow her on Twitter: Twitter.com/ClaudiaYoga